This book is dedicated to my patients.
Thank you for trusting me with your smile.

DENTAL IMPLANTS
Idea Section 2

The **WONDER**
of **DENTAL IMPLANTS** . 19

REASONS TO REPLACE
LOST TEETH 27

DENTAL IMPLANT
Checklist 36

AFTER
SURGERY. 40

Disclaimer
This book was written for informational purposes only. It is meant to provide general background information for patients and to serve as an educational tool or conversation starter. The examples and pictures in this book should not be taken as medical or dental advice. Every person is different and requires a personalized treatment plan from a licensed dentist. Neither the publisher nor the author shall be liable for any damages that result from unsuccessful dental treatment. Note that some of the information in this book may be incorrect or out of date.

DENTAL IMPLANTS
Idea Section

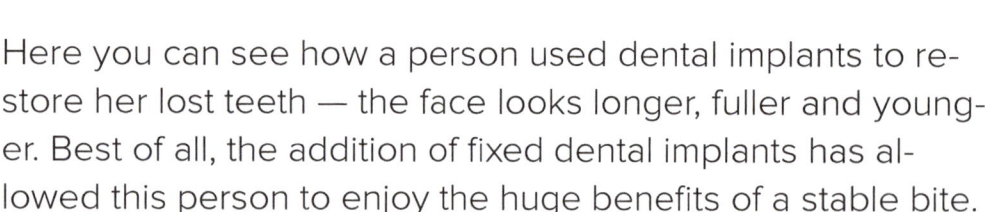

Idea 1: Completely replace all top teeth

Here you can see how a person used dental implants to restore her lost teeth — the face looks longer, fuller and younger. Best of all, the addition of fixed dental implants has allowed this person to enjoy the huge benefits of a stable bite.

Interesting side note: Before the patient came in for dental implant therapy, she had much shorter smaller teeth. Because all of her top teeth were being replaced, her teeth could be made much larger and more beautiful. The size of the teeth was worked out with a removable denture that served as her temporary teeth while the dental implants healed underneath

For most cases where all the upper teeth are being replaced with dental implant supported crowns, a removable denture is often necessary. This denture temporarily provides teeth while dental implants heal underneath. It also helps to provide guidance in terms of the final outcome since a lot of the major issues can be settled using a denture (cosmetic appearance, size of teeth, color of teeth etc.)

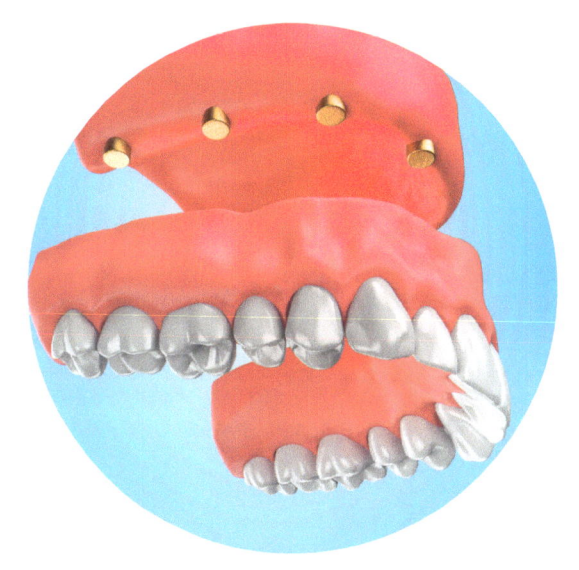

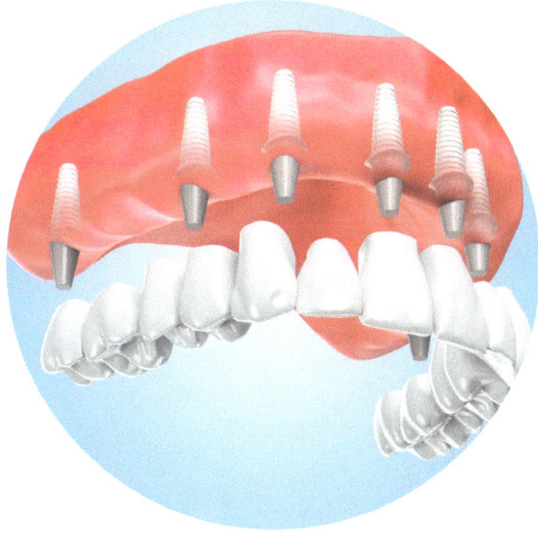

Creating the smile above was made possible using dental implants. Often, the 12 to 14 teeth being placed are split into 3 different sections. These sections are back right teeth, back left teeth and front teeth. The way that it is actually split up depends on patient's bone quality and the number of teeth being replaced. Every case is highly individualized and requires careful planning.

In cases where dental implants are not ideally placed or compromised, it may be necessary to create a single bridge of 12 to 14 teeth rather than split it up into sections. This concept of "splinting" or connecting implants together takes advantage of a concept called "cross arch stabilization" which pretty much means even force distribution across all teeth.

Idea 2:
Completely replace all bottom teeth

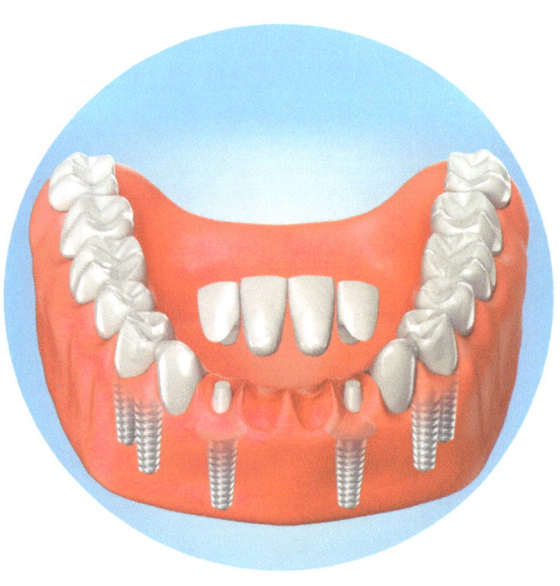

Similarly to top teeth, implant supported bottom teeth are also often split into several bridges so that it is easier to fabricate. Sometimes they are all connected together to improve dental implant success rate.

In the photo below, the patient has 3 implant — supported bridges replacing all of his bottom teeth. 7 Dental implants were used to support 12 teeth. The patient decided to use a removable denture to replace the top teeth.

Interesting story: After wearing the denture for several years, the patient continually commented how much more comfortable fixed implant supported teeth were than plastic removable teeth (dentures). After some time, the patient decided to go through dental implant therapy to replace his top teeth as well.

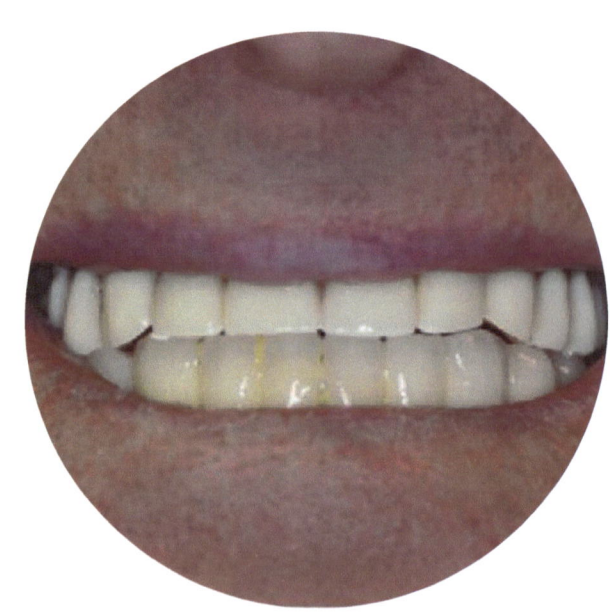

Idea 3:
Front teeth fixed,
back teeth removable

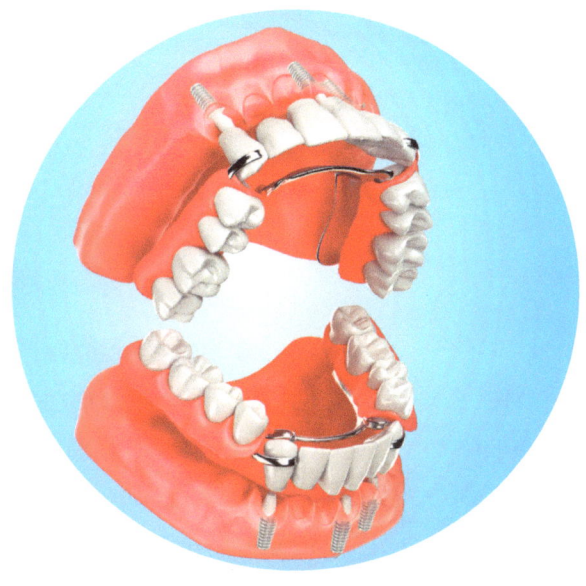

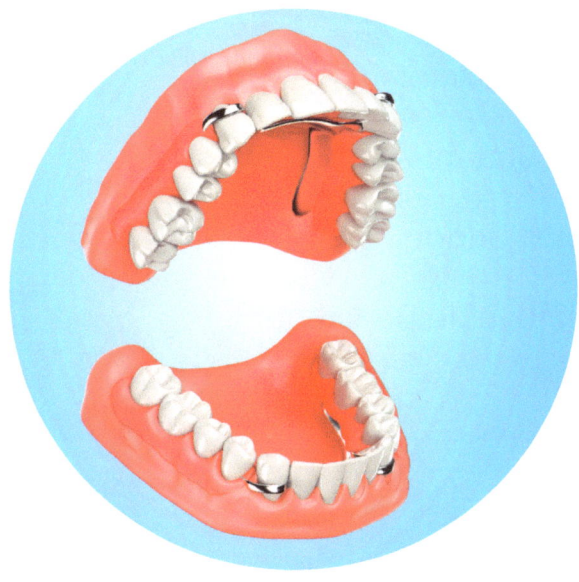

This is an excellent option for those people who want to have fixed front teeth and removable back teeth. In this case, 3 dental implants are used to support 6 front teeth on both the top and the bottom. A small removable partial denture replaces back chewing teeth. In this option, even when you take off your dentures, your front teeth remain which helps to maintain facial dimensions and is generally more comfortable.

Requires:

- 3 dental implants

- 3 abutments

- 6 unit bridge

- Removable partial denture

Idea 4:
8 fixed teeth front, back teeth removable

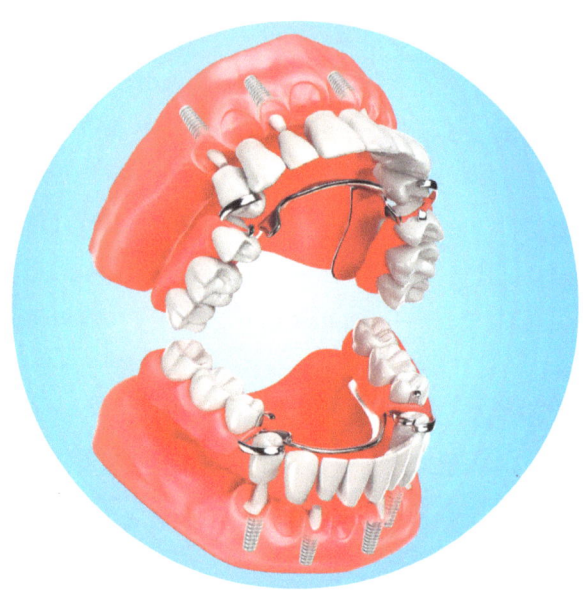

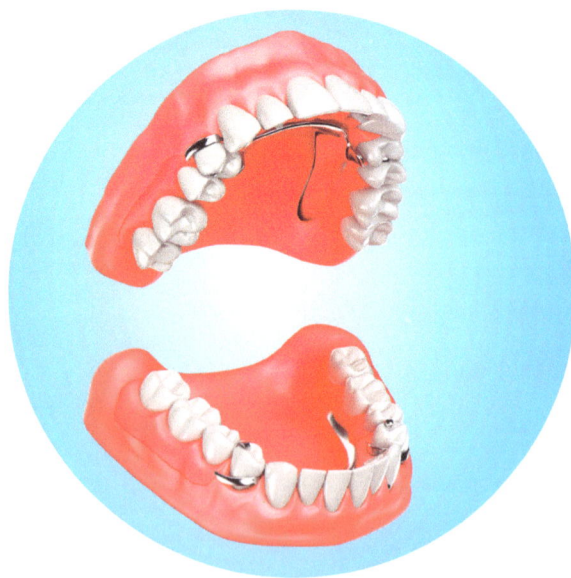

This option gives you 8 fixed teeth. That's the six front teeth and 2 back teeth. While not enough to chew completely, it provides a nice balance of fixed teeth to denture teeth.

Requires:

- 4 dental implants

- 4 abutments

- 8 unit bridge

- Removable partial denture

Idea 5:
10 fixed teeth front, small section of back teeth removable

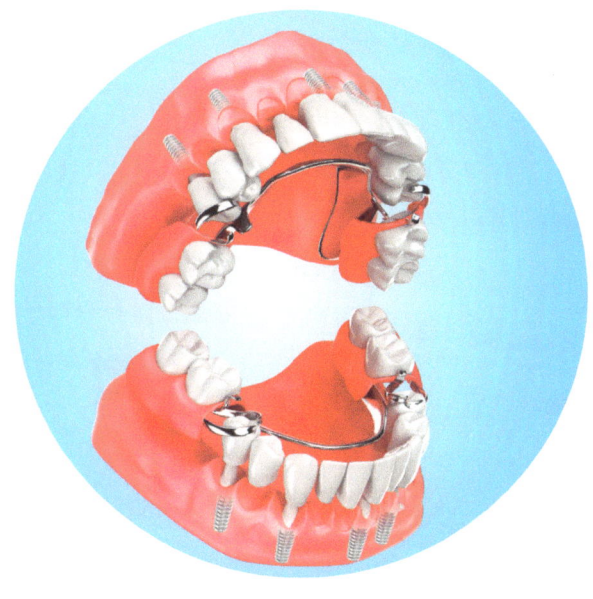

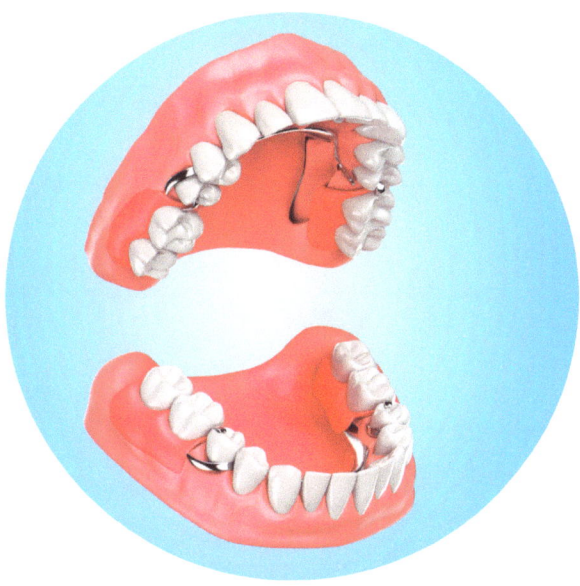

This is an option that provides the least amount of teeth necessary to chew well. Based on several studies, 10 teeth on top and bottom is enough to chew without needing a partial denture. For those who want a full set of teeth, a small partial is helpful.

Requires:

- 5 dental implants

- 5 abutments

- 10 unit bridge

- Optional: removable partial denture

Idea 6:
Completely fixed top and bottom teeth

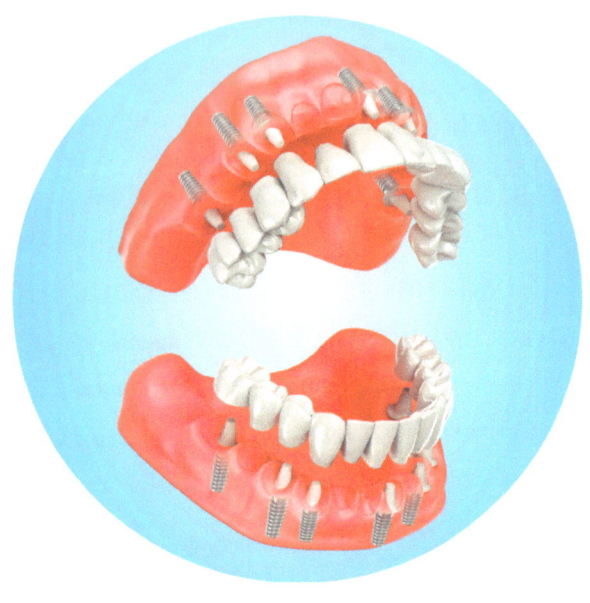

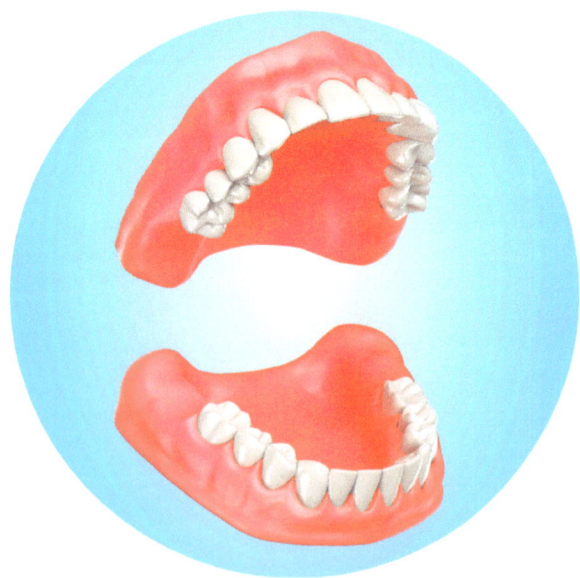

Widely considered the best option by most dental professionals. A fixed set of teeth on 7 to 8 dental implants is as natural and comfortable as dental technology allows. Crowns are small, smooth and effective at chewing food. This option is usually the easiest to get used to and often the most cosmetically pleasing.

Requires:

- 7 to 8 implants

- 7 to 8 abutments

- 12–14 crowns

Idea 7: Make your top denture more comfortable

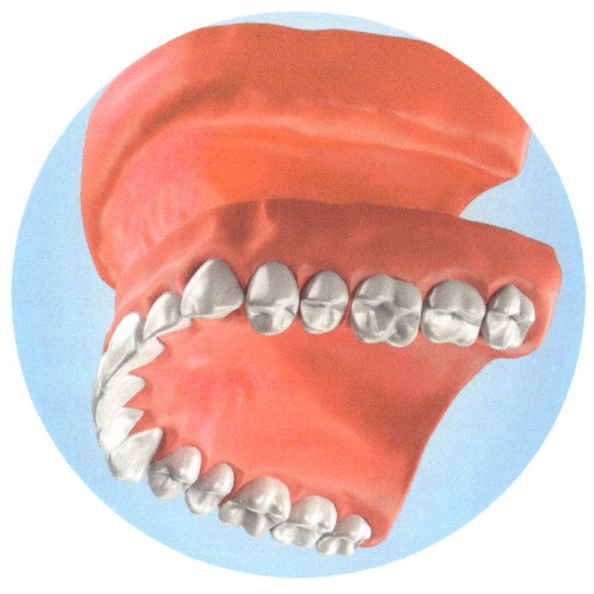

A complete removable top denture can often be comfortable. This is especially true because well made upper dentures usually boast powerful suction to the palate and stay in place during eating. The biggest problem with removable upper dentures is that they completely cover the palate which decreases a person's sense of taste and food temperature. It's also a major issue for people who have a sensitive gag reflex

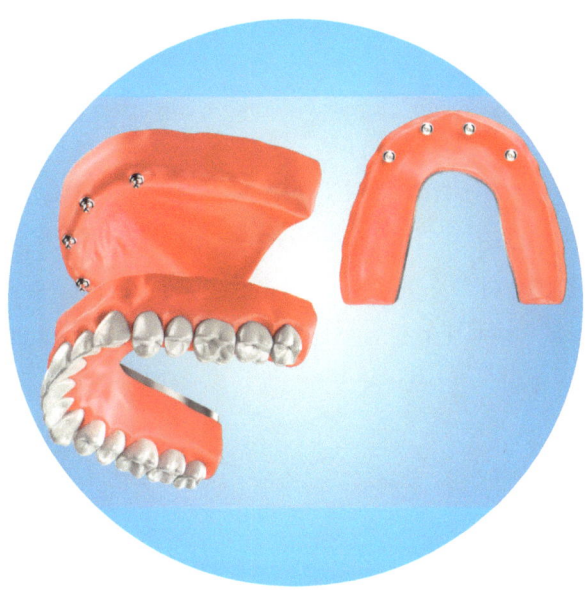

A complete removable top denture can often be comfortable. This is especially true because well made upper dentures usually boast powerful suction to the palate and stay in place during eating. The biggest problem with removable upper dentures is that they completely cover the palate which decreases a person's sense of taste and food temperature. It's also a major issue for people who have a sensitive gag reflex

Idea 8: Make your bottom denture more stable

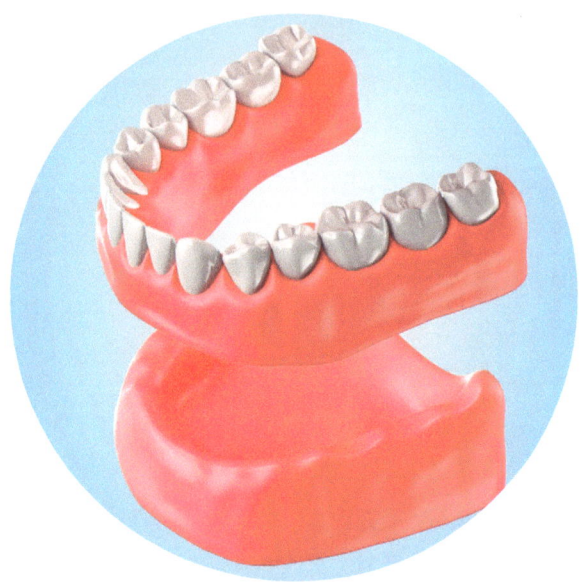

Lower complete dentures are notoriously the least accepted by patients. Unlike upper dentures which boast suction and usually stay in place, lower dentures are often loose and are dislodged easily by the tongue during chewing and eating.

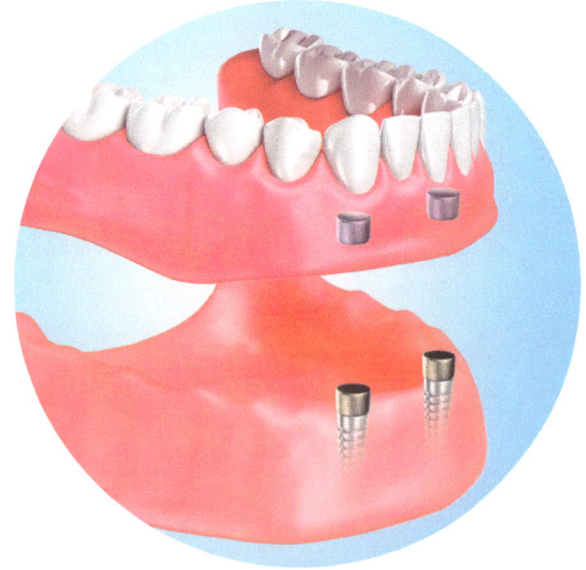

Two dental implants placed in the front of the mouth make a huge difference for patients with lower dentures. It ensures that the denture stays in place when you speak and chew.

Idea 9:
Replace A Single tooth

Front tooth

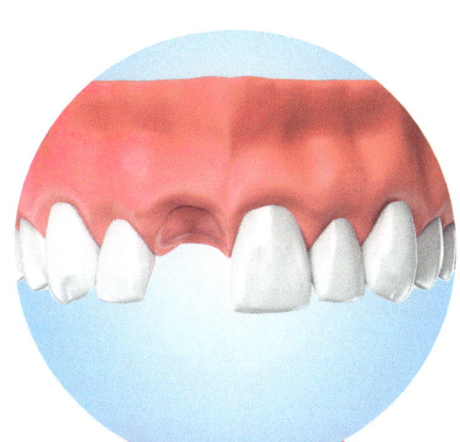

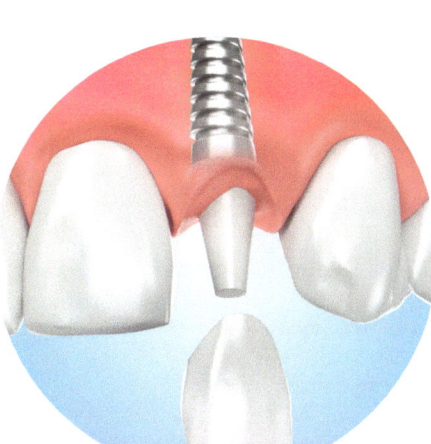

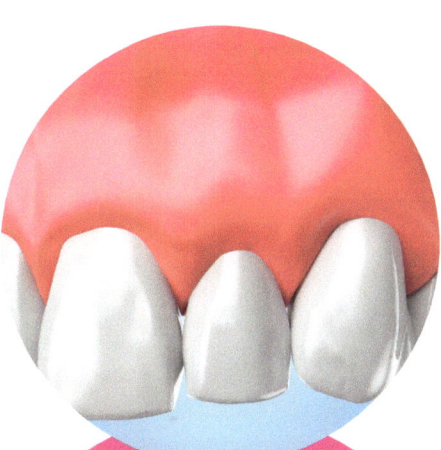

If you are missing a single tooth and the remaining teeth are completely healthy, dental implant therapy is a no brainer. It's the most conservative and durable approach to tooth replacement.

Using a dental implant to replace a single tooth allows surrounding teeth to remain untouched. When done properly, the results can be very natural and cosmetically pleasing.

A dental implant crown can look and feel natural.

Idea 10:
Sinus lift and bone graft

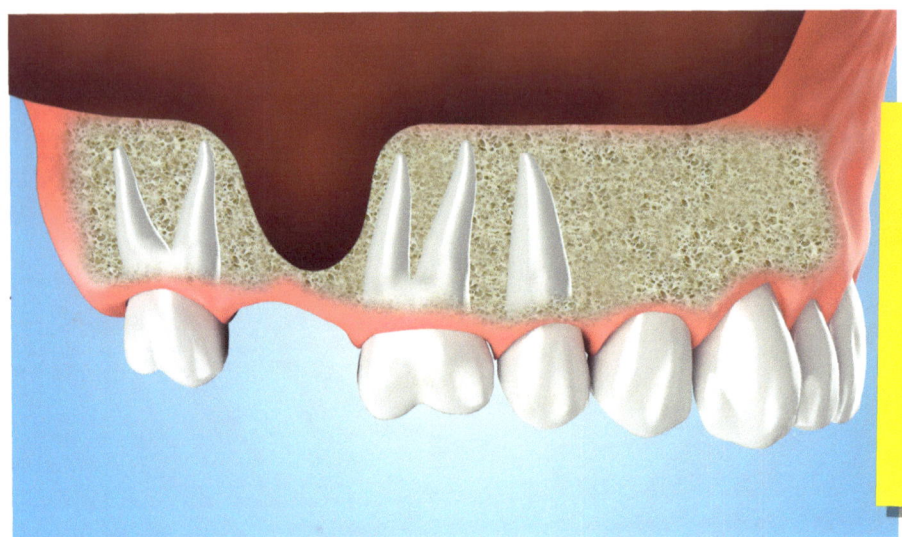

Here you can see a very common scenario: not enough bone to place a dental implant. With today's bone grafting techniques, this is no longer a problem.

By lifting the sinus and putting in bone grafting material, the body can naturally grow more bone and allow for the placement of a dental implant.

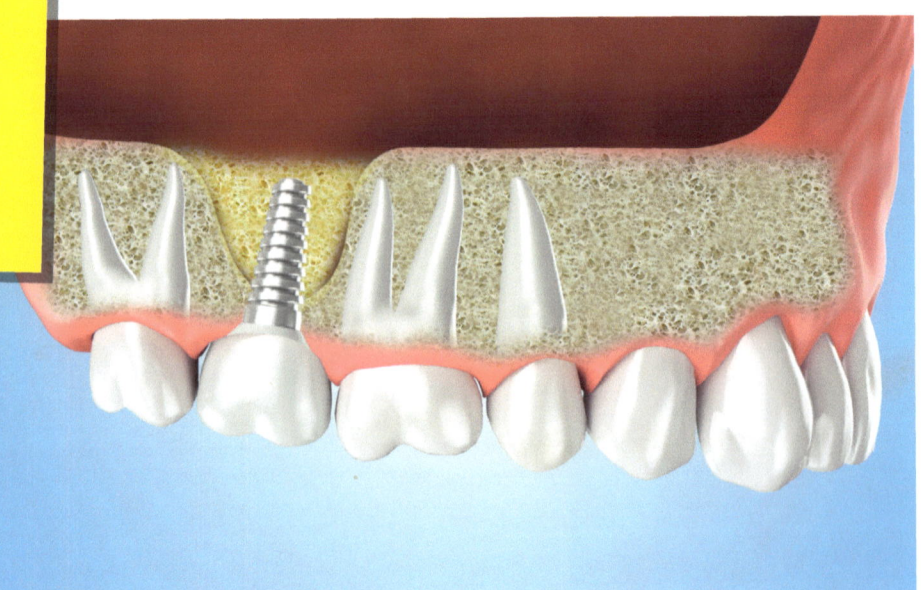

Idea 11:
Replace a small section of teeth with a dental implant supported bridge

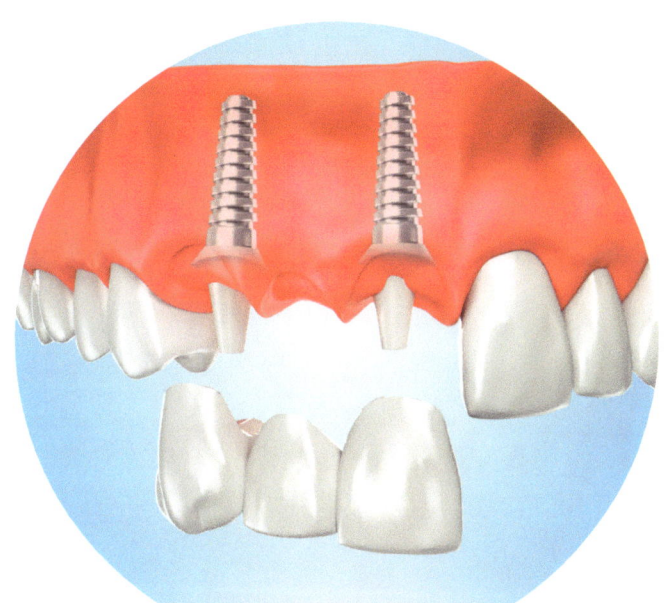

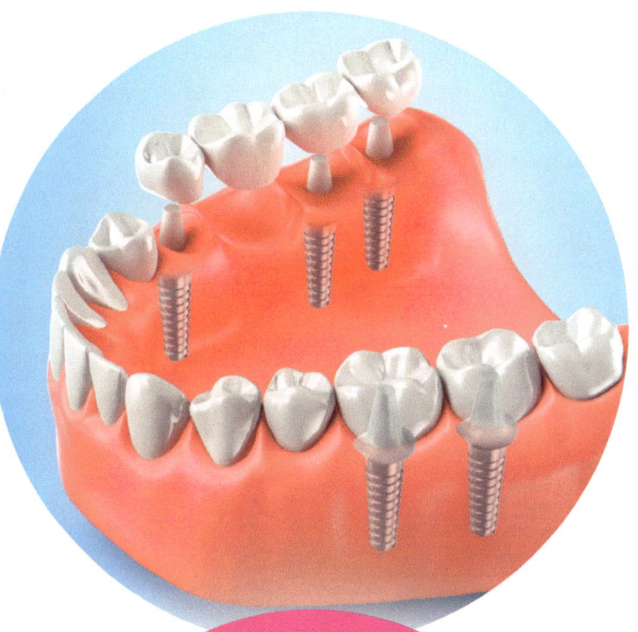

Here you can see that several front teeth are missing. In this case two dental implants can actually replace 3 total teeth.

Here a patient is missing several back teeth. On the right side, 3 dental implants are used to support a bridge of 4 teeth. On the left, two dental implants replace two teeth.

Idea 12:
One dental implant to support a partial denture

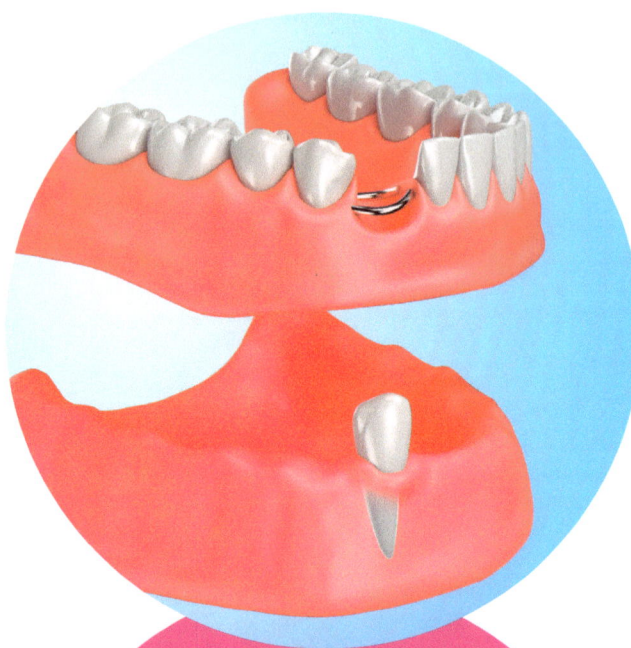

Here you can see a situation where a patient has just one tooth left on the bottom. Often, having just one tooth doesn't provide enough support for a large lower partial denture. In this case it's advisable to add a single dental implant to the other side.

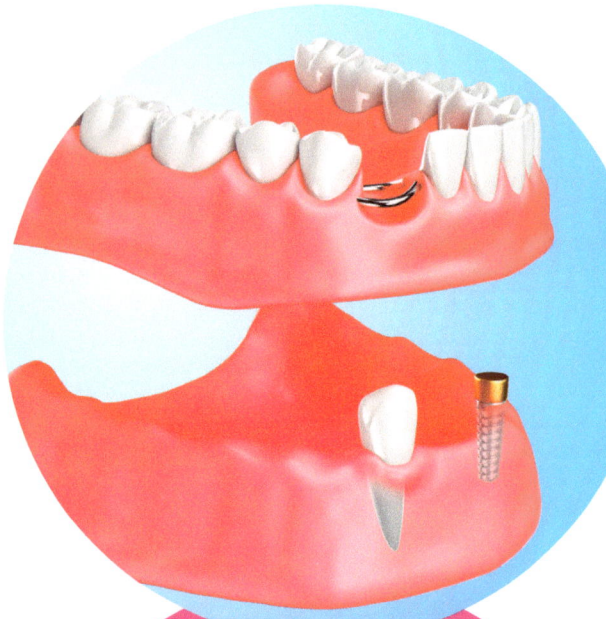

Here is the same patient after the addition of a dental implant. Now the partial denture has far more support and is likely to be more secure and comfortable. Eventually, if the other natural tooth becomes loose, another implant may be needed to ensure patient's comfort.

Idea 13:
Immediate placement
of implant and temporary crown

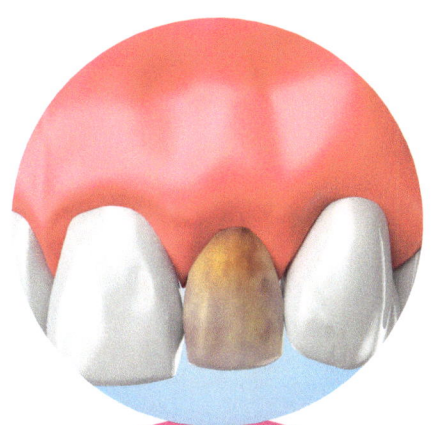

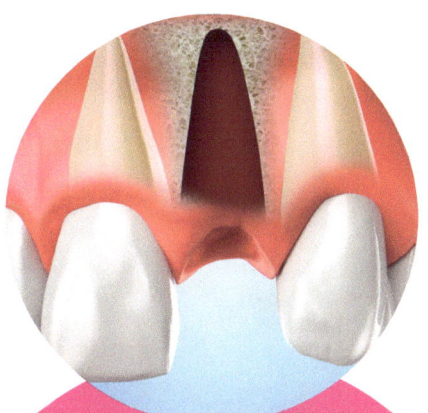

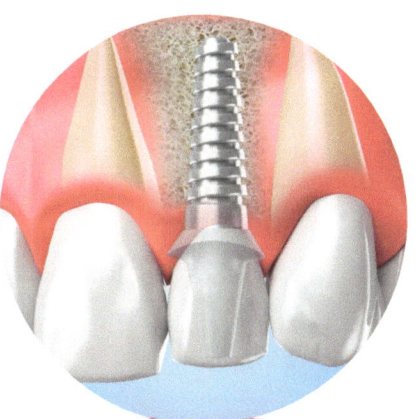

Here you can see that several front teeth are missing. In this case two dental implants can actually replace 3 total teeth.

Immediately after placement, an abutment can be placed and temporary crown placed on top. Though it cannot be used to bite into food, it provides a cosmetic cover so that you can continue to smile confidently through daily life.

Often, a surgeon can gently remove the broken tooth and place a dental implant into the same location.

Idea 14:
Make your denture smaller and more comfortable

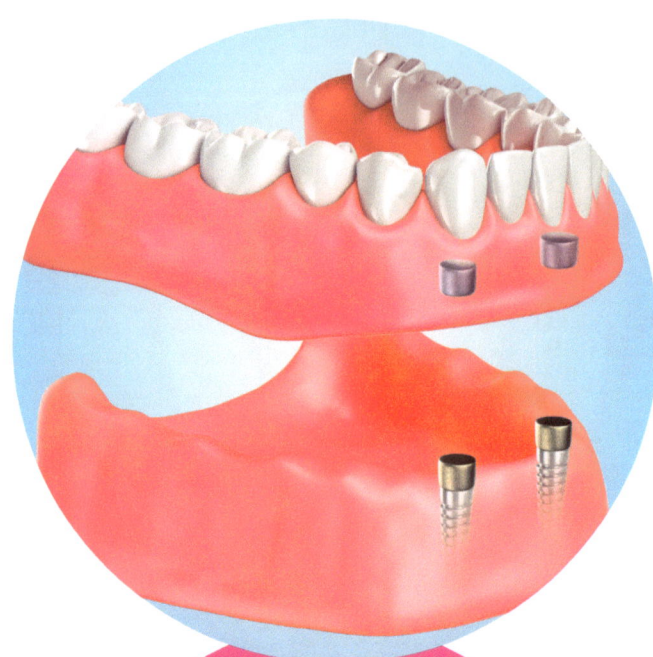

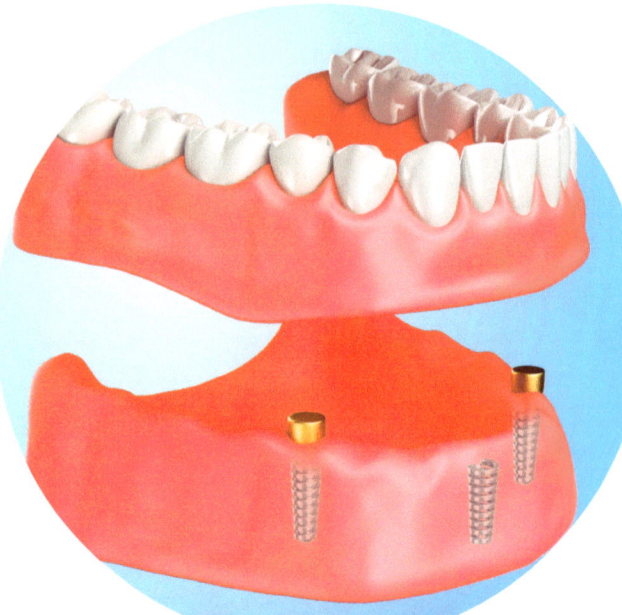

This patient started with a removable denture on the bottom supported by 2 dental implants with locator attachments.

Then the patient decided he wants his lower front teeth to be fixed rather than removable. A dental implant is placed between these two implants and the patient continues to wear the denture as this implant integrates for a few months.

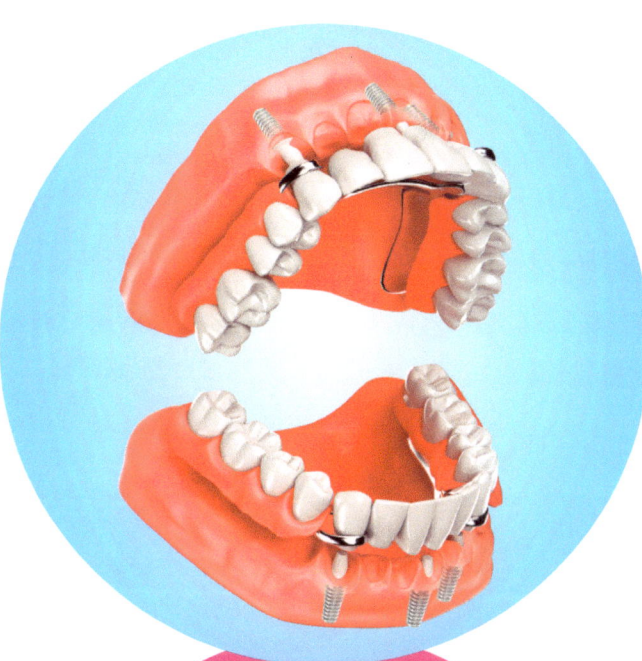

Once the implant has successfully integrated, the golden locators are unscrewed and replaced with abutments and a bridge of 6 teeth. These lower front teeth are fixed. To replace the missing back teeth, a small partial denture is made.

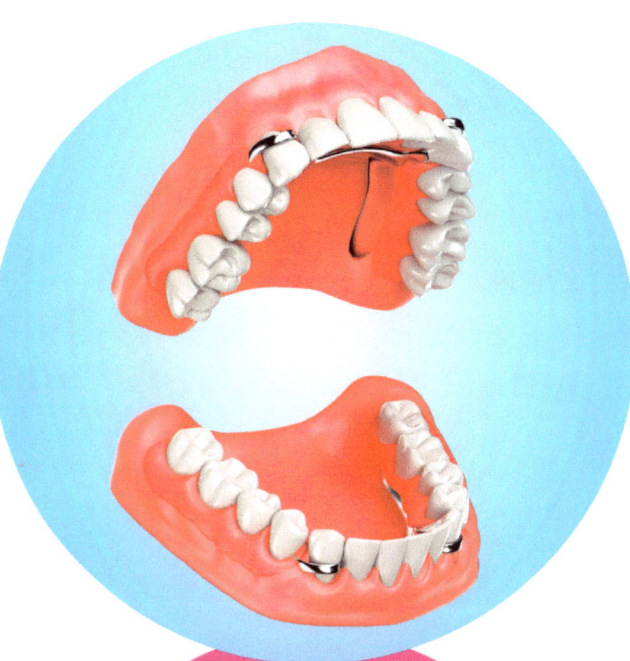

Here is the finished result: A well-fitting partial denture to replace back chewing teeth and a fixed 6 unit bridge to replace the front teeth.

Idea 15:
Go from removable teeth to fixed teeth

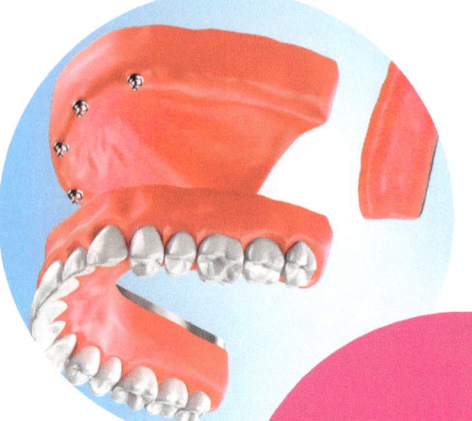

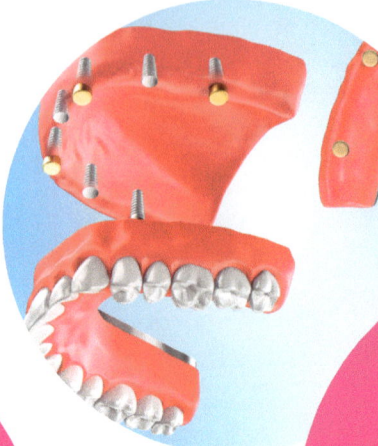

This patient started out with an implant supported upper denture and then decided that she wants fixed (non removable) teeth.

Three dental implants are placed into the correct positions and the patient continues to wear the denture as the new implants integrate underneath. This patient's life remains unchanged while the implants heal.

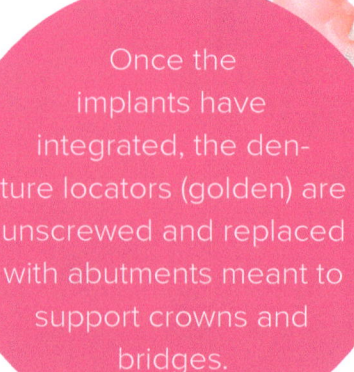

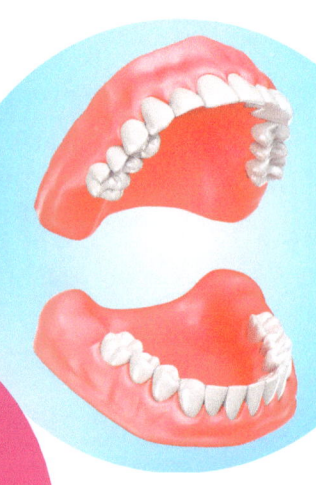

Once the implants have integrated, the denture locators (golden) are unscrewed and replaced with abutments meant to support crowns and bridges.

Here you can see the finished result. This patient replaced her removable denture with fixed teeth that never have to come out and are more comfortable.

the WONDER OF Dental Implants

Dental implants — An accidental discovery!

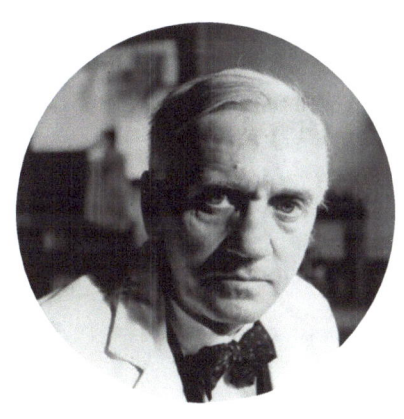

Sir Alexander Fleming

Sir Alexander Fleming, a Scottish biologist, accidentally discovered penicillin — which has forever changed the way we treat bacterial infection. Similarly, dental implants were discovered by accident. Dr. Branemark, a Swedish physician, was doing experiments on bone healing using specially designed titanium tubes implanted into rabbits. At the end of an experiment — when he went to take the tubes out of the rabbits, he realized that he couldn't. Bone had fused with the titanium tube and "Osseointegrated." This began a journey that ended up in the introduction of dental implants and changed dentistry forever.

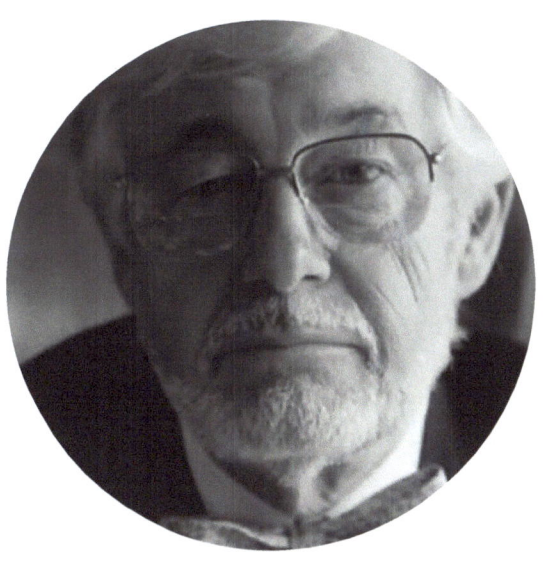

Dr. Branemark

REASONS
to LOVE
Dental Implants

The odds are in your favor

The widespread popularity of dental implants can be linked to their predictability. Overall, dental implant success rate has been documented as 98%. Other popular figures to help explain success rate are 99% success in the mandible or bottom jaws and 95% in the top jaws or maxilla.

These are truly great odds which explain why in 2006 alone, more than 5 million dental implants were placed in the United States. In fact, the dental implant market is projected to reach 5 billion by 2018. In other words, dental implants are here to stay and will only become more popular as time goes on.

The highest value treatment option

When patients are offered dental implant therapy to treat tooth loss, they often question if it's worth the cost. However, they are often not thinking long term. Consider this:

- A traditional bridge to replace one tooth lasts an average of 10 years before failing.

- Only 60% of removable partial dentures survive after 4 years and the tooth that supports the clasps is often lost after 10 years (leading to more tooth loss).

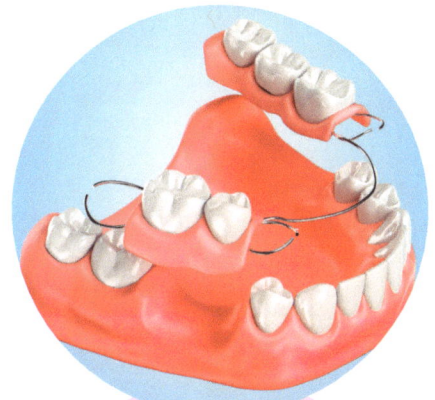

Removable Denture

40% of removable dentures fail after 4 years.

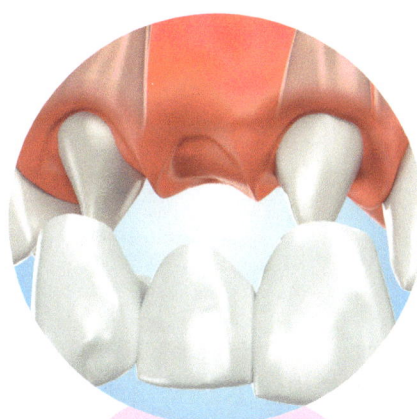

Dental bridges on teeth last an average of 10 years before failing.

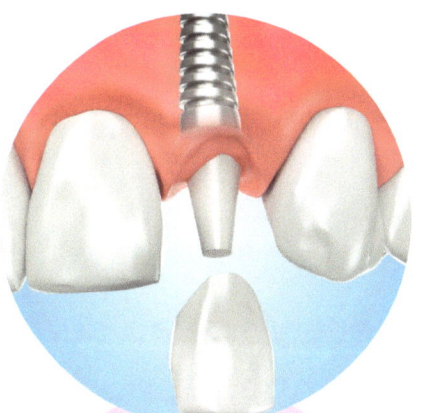

A single implant and crown has a 97% success rate after 10 years.

Now consider recent evidence about dental implant crowns and bridges: A single implant and crown has a success rate of 97% after 10 years. A bridge using dental implants has a survival rate of 87% after 10 years. While conventional tooth replacement options may seem "cheaper," dental implant therapy is usually a higher value and more predictable option in the long run.

Live a better life

Study after study confirms that in the vast majority of cases, people who undergo dental implant therapy to treat tooth loss report higher quality of life score than those who don't. This applies to both denture patients who add dental implants to increase denture stability and to patients who opt for fixed (non — removable) bridges using dental implants.

Here you can see how adding implant supported crowns relieves pressure from the remaining teeth. By adding these 6 teeth, heavy forces that occur during chewing are more evenly distributed. Maintaining a stable bite is an important part of saving remaining natural teeth.

It's no secret that the best teeth are those made by nature rather than a dentist. While it's not always possible to maintain your natural teeth, dental implants give us the opportunity to hold onto them as long as possible. Replacing lost teeth with dental implants ensures that chewing forces are distributed evenly. It also ensures a stable bite.

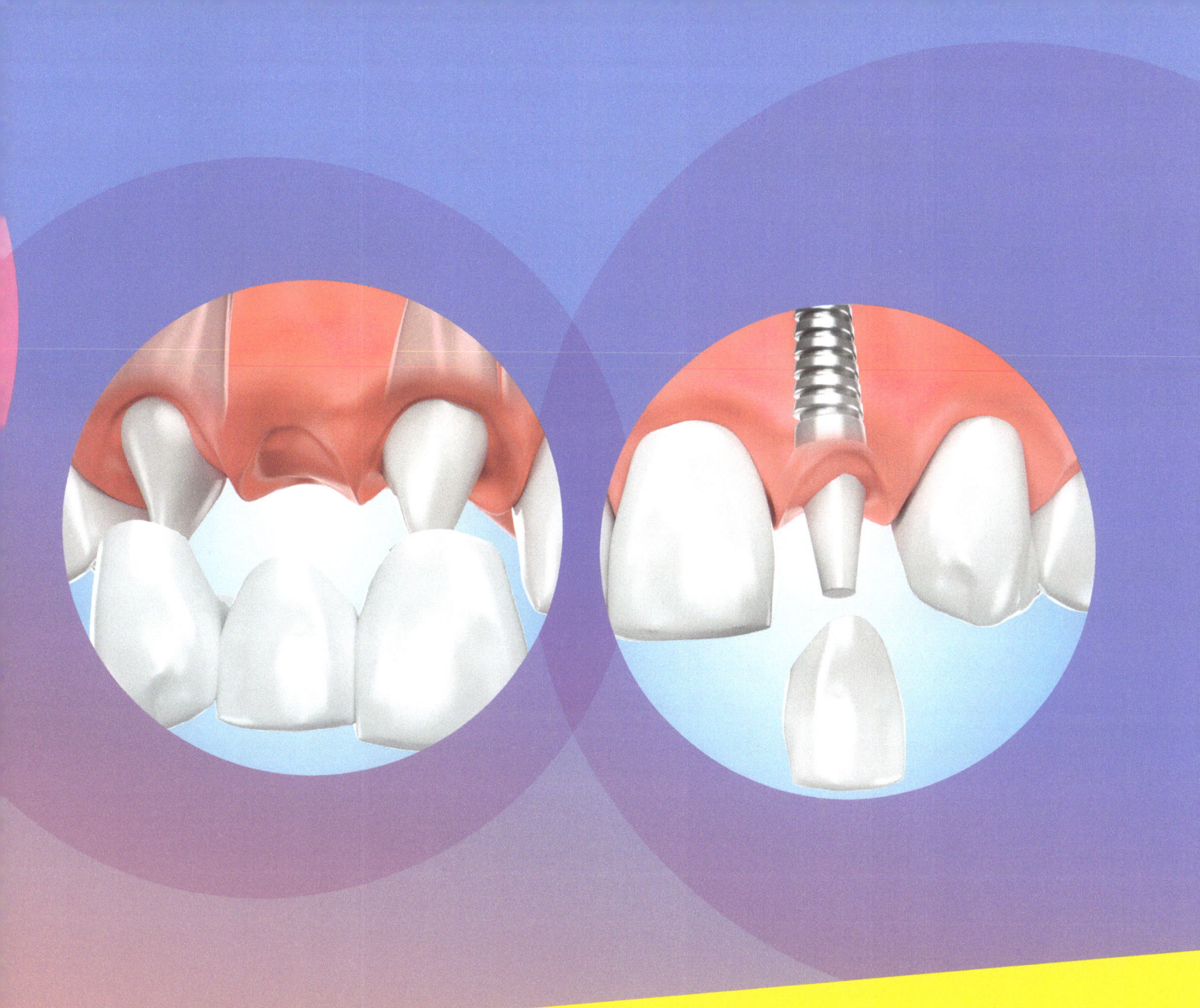

Don't mess with nature!

A traditional dental bridge on teeth requires shaving of tooth structure and often creates hygiene issues. Notice how much tooth must be trimmed to accommodate a bridge. In this case, a dental implant supported crown is the obvious and conservative choice. By using a dental implant, the neighboring teeth are left untouched and can easily be flossed.

Unless a tooth has received root canal therapy or is already broken down, shaving it down just to allow a bridge to be put on top is aggressive and wasteful.

No cavities ever again!

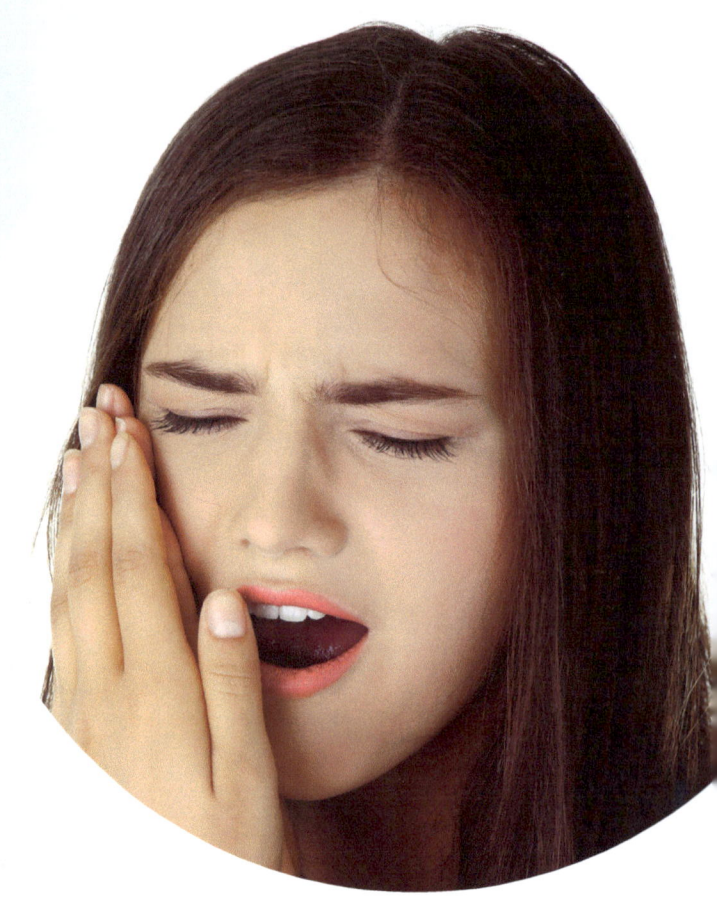

Tooth sensitivity and root canals — a common problem with teeth — is not something you have to worry about with dental implants. That's because dental implants can't decay and have no nerve endings.

Because dental implants are made out of titanium, they never decay. The bugs that cause decay of teeth can wreak havoc on a person's mouth. In fact, decay is often the reason behind failure of tooth supported crowns and bridges. Decay in natural teeth can lead to root canals, tooth sensitivity and even the need for extraction.

Here you can see how bacteria can cause a tooth to decay but has little effect on the dental implant. While dental implants are susceptible to gum disease (periodontitis), dental caries (cavities) are usually not a major concern in implant dentistry.

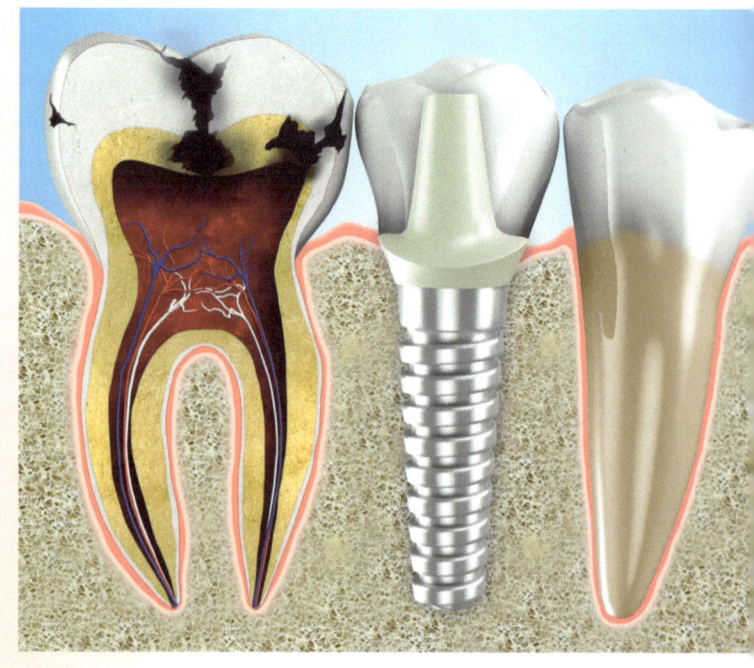

Keep your teeth where they belong — in your mouth!

Dental implants help to keep teeth where they belong — in your mouth. The fear of having teeth fall out can cause anxiety and can affect a person's self image. Using dental implants to help stabilize removable dentures can make a big difference in a patient's comfort level. Using them to retain fixed crowns and bridges is the closest thing there is to having natural teeth.

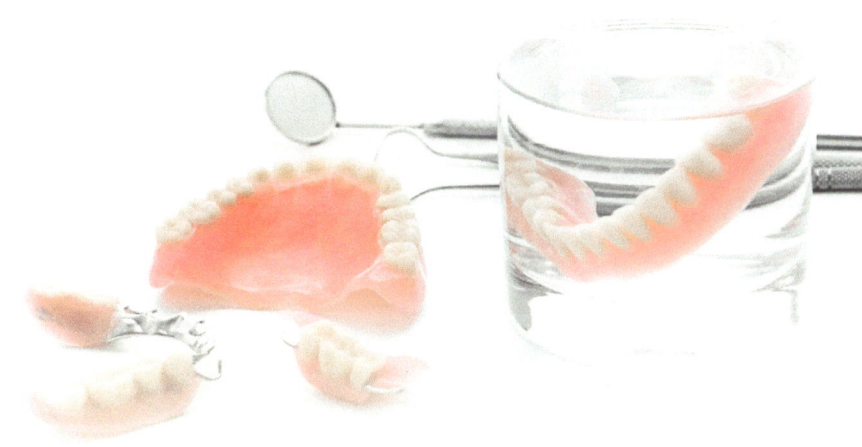

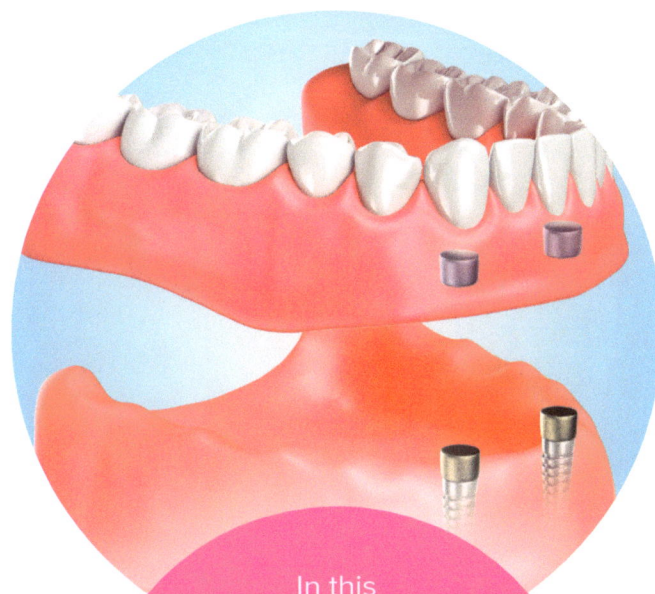

In this scenario, a person can have peace of mind that their lower denture is not going to fall out while talking or eating. Just 2 dental implants make a huge difference.

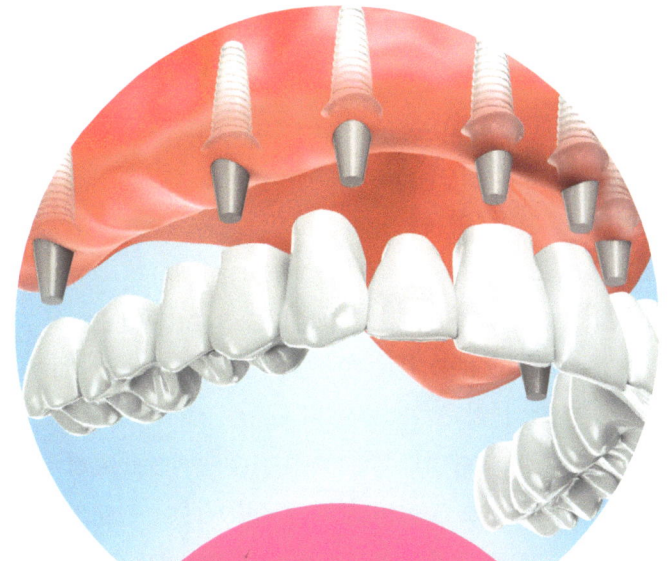

Here you can see six dental implants supporting 3 fixed bridges. In this case, the patient doesn't have to take anything out of their mouth at any point. It's as close to natural teeth as it gets.

As close as it gets to natural teeth

A dental implant is as close to a natural tooth as it gets in terms of comfort and durability. While healthy natural teeth are still better than implants, nothing in dental therapy comes as close to mimicking natural teeth as dental implants. This allows people to have a very comfortable and beautiful set of teeth even if natural teeth have been lost.

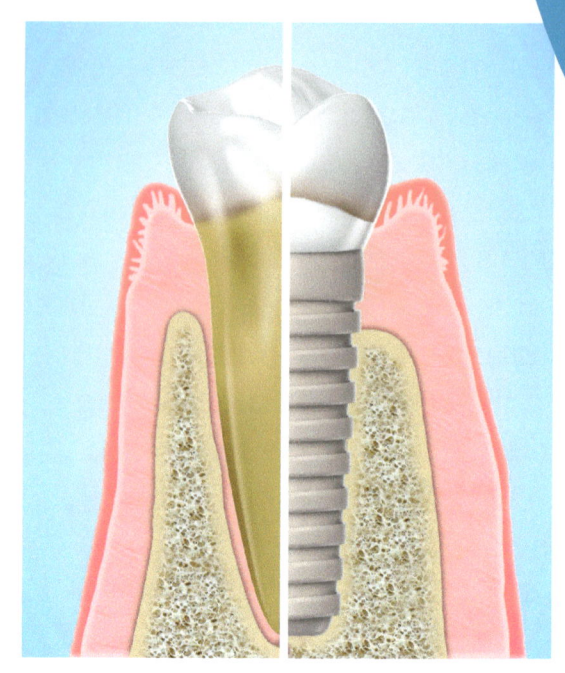

Does your bite practice self defense?

In dentistry, there is a concept known as a self-defending bite. This generally means that there are enough teeth to bite and chew. When we eat, the front teeth known as the incisors bite into food and then the back teeth chew the food up. If there aren't enough teeth, remaining teeth become overloaded and the bite begins to collapse. Using dental implants, an ideal amount of teeth can be placed so that the balance between biting and chewing teeth remains equal and the bite defends itself from heavy chewing forces. Only dental implants can do this in a conservative and predictable way.

REASONS
to replace
Lost Teeth

Don't Lose Face

Teeth and dental implants do more than just help to chew. They also stimulate the surrounding bone and maintain the height and contours of our face. Here you can see how having a full set of teeth helps to ensure healthy bone and facial appearance.

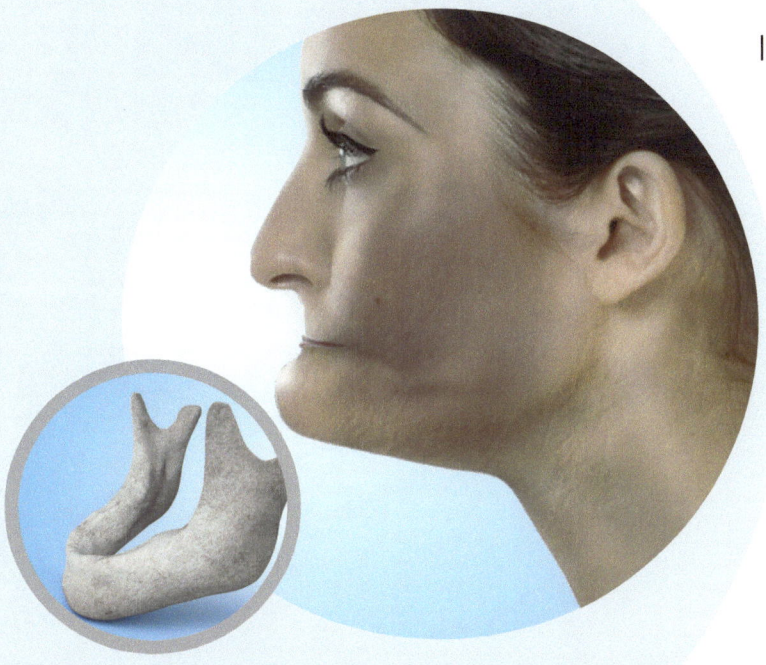

If teeth are lost and not replaced with dental implants, the bone that usually supports them gradually disappears. As a result, the bite begins to collapse and this affects the length of a person's face as well as the way the cheeks and lips appear — most often the appearance of old age is associated with caved in lips and cheeks. Generally, early tooth loss without permanent replacement causes people to look older.

You don't have to go to the gym for maintenance of facial muscles

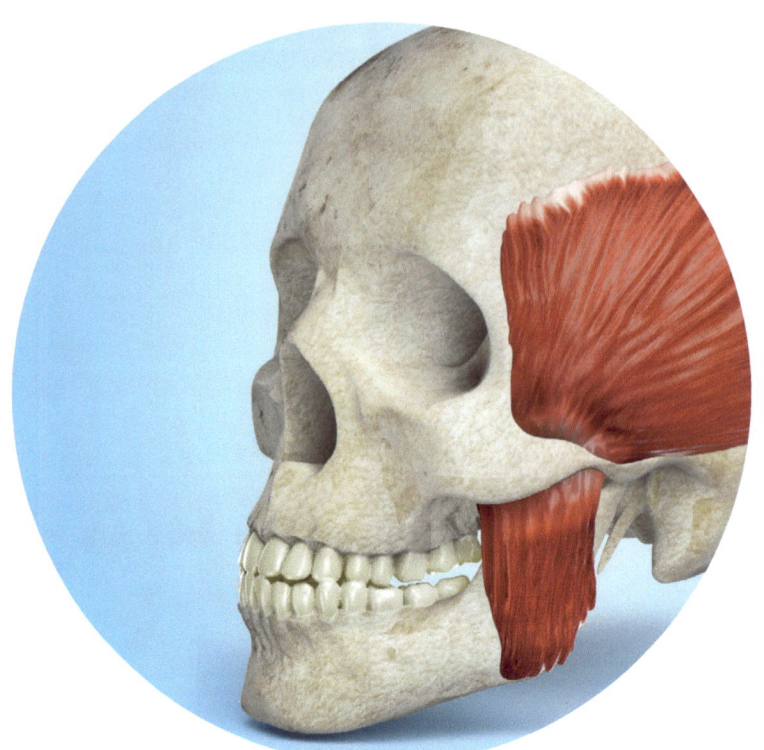

When it comes to the muscles of the face, you don't have to be at the gym to maintain them. What's troubling though is that facial muscles can actually become weaker if enough fixed teeth are not maintained.

Several studies have suggested that denture wearers only have about ¼ to 1/5 of the bite strength compared to people with fixed dental implants or natural teeth. They often have to chew 7 times harder to process the same food and also have chewing muscles that are weaker. This is why it is thought that denture wearers may avoid hard nutritious foods that are difficult to chew. The result is a eating a soft and less nutritious diet that may lead to an array of health problems.

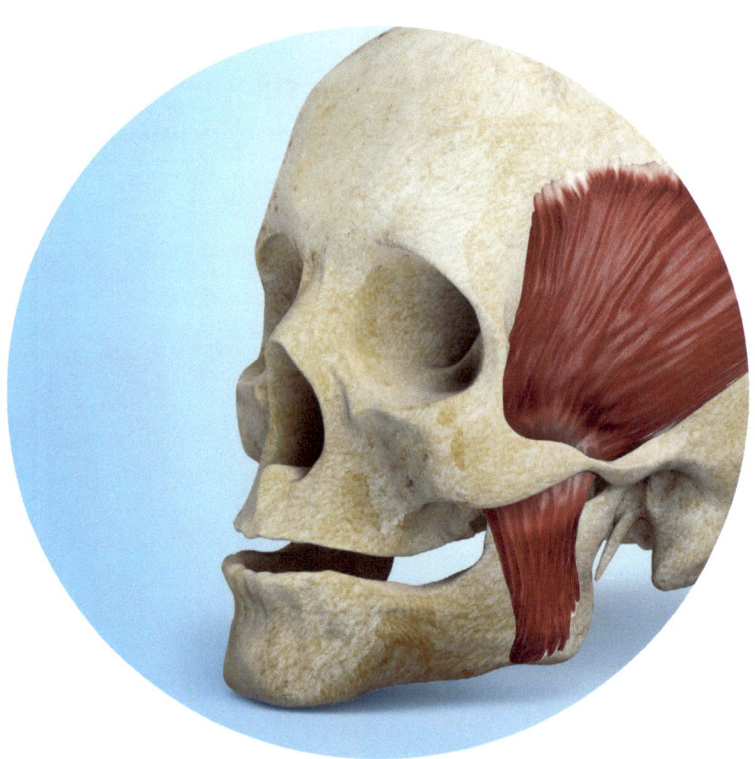

Enough is Enough!

Based on several studies, the minimum number of teeth a person needs to chew well is 20 — that is 10 on the top and 10 on the bottom. The number of teeth usually recommended to help ensure optimal chewing is 12 on the top and 12 on the bottom — which is 24 in all.

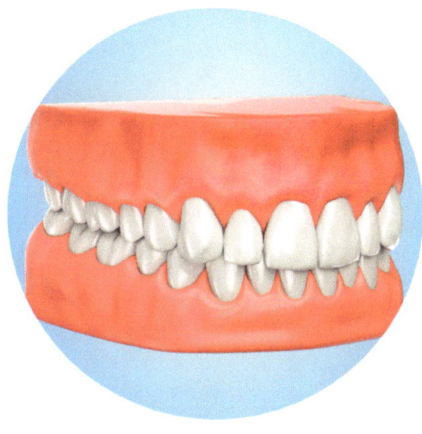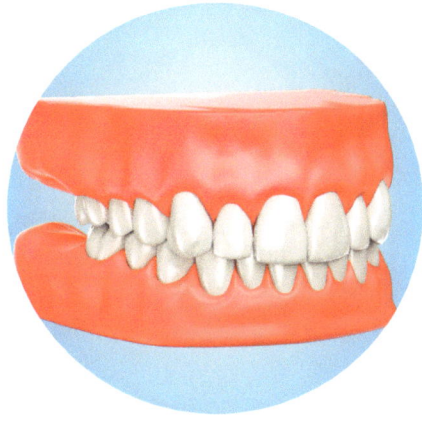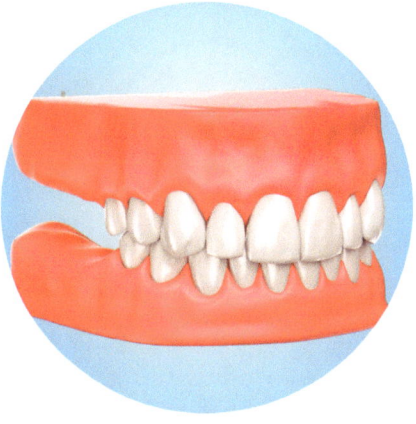

The maximum number of teeth for any human is 32 but the 3rd molars are often taken out so many people end up with a total of 28 total teeth if all their teeth are perfectly healthy.

Here you can see a more optimal number of teeth. This is a total of 24 teeth and replaces about 95% of chewing ability.

Here you can see the minimum number of teeth necessary to chew food well. It shows 10 teeth on the top and 10 teeth on the bottom. Though this is considered enough teeth by some studies, many patients find out that they need an additional tooth on each side for complete satisfaction.

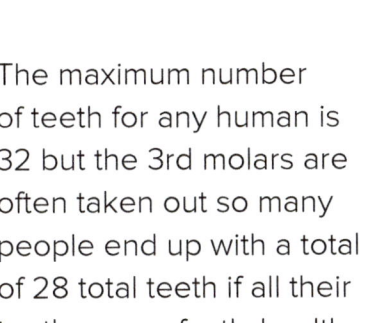

A Deadly Diet

Evidence shows that people who don't have enough teeth make poor food choices. This may be because it's much harder to chew and process healthy foods like fruits and vegetables. Crunchy food high in fiber, carotene and antioxidants is often replaced with food that is higher in fat and artery clogging cholesterol. Poor nutrition has drastic consequences including obesity, heart disease and gastrointestinal problems.

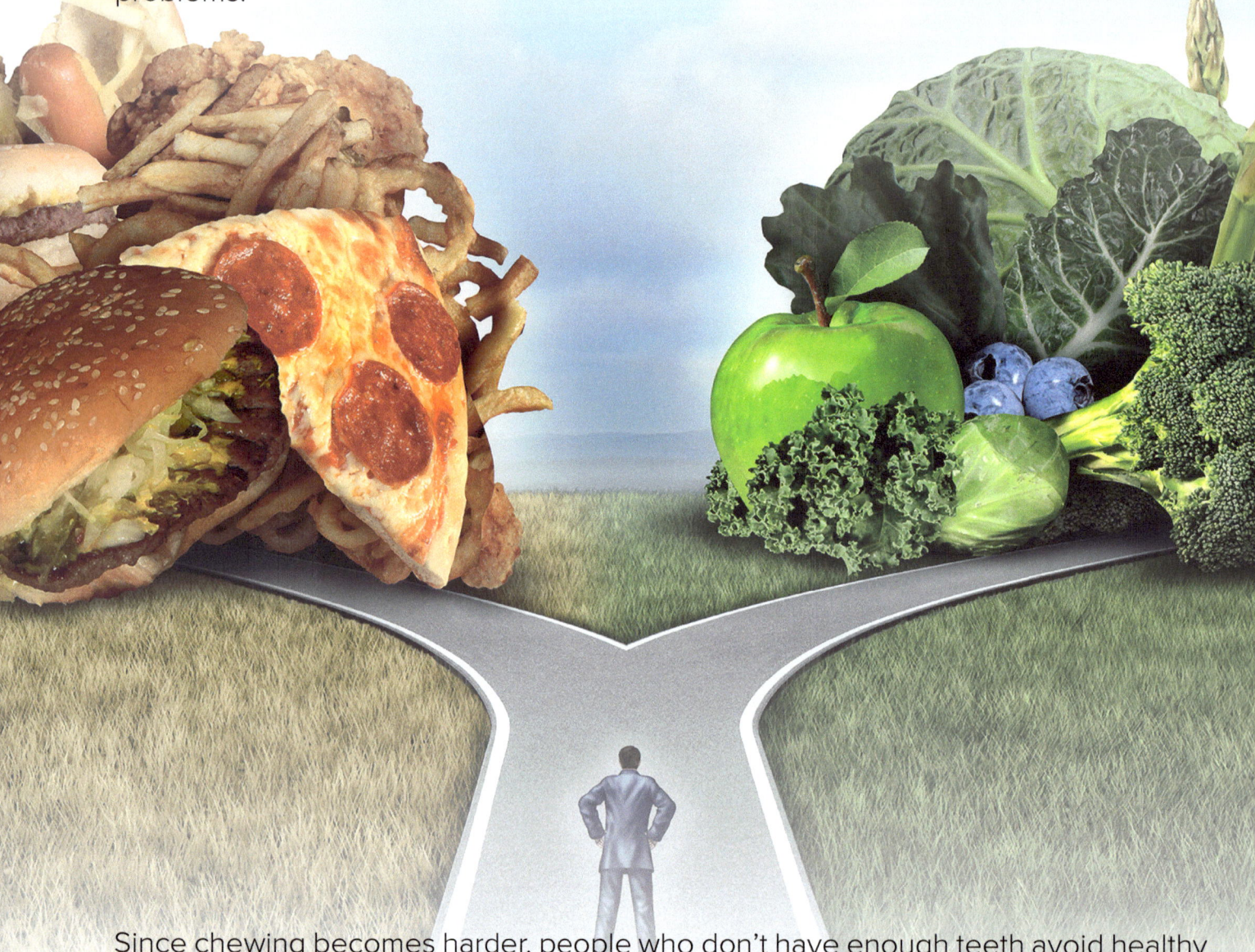

Since chewing becomes harder, people who don't have enough teeth avoid healthy foods high in fiber, carotene and antioxidants like certain fruits and vegetables. Many times these decisions happen without the person even realizing that they are making food choices based on chewing difficulty.

The Dreaded "C Word"

Many people don't realize that digestion begins in the mouth. Without enough teeth to properly chew and process food, the entire digestive system suffers. New evidence points out that tooth loss may contribute to chronic inflammation of the digestive system. This can lead to painful ulcers of the stomach and small intestine — something that further complicates the ability to make healthy food choices. In extreme cases, tooth loss has even been suggested to play a role in pancreatic and gastrointestinal cancer.

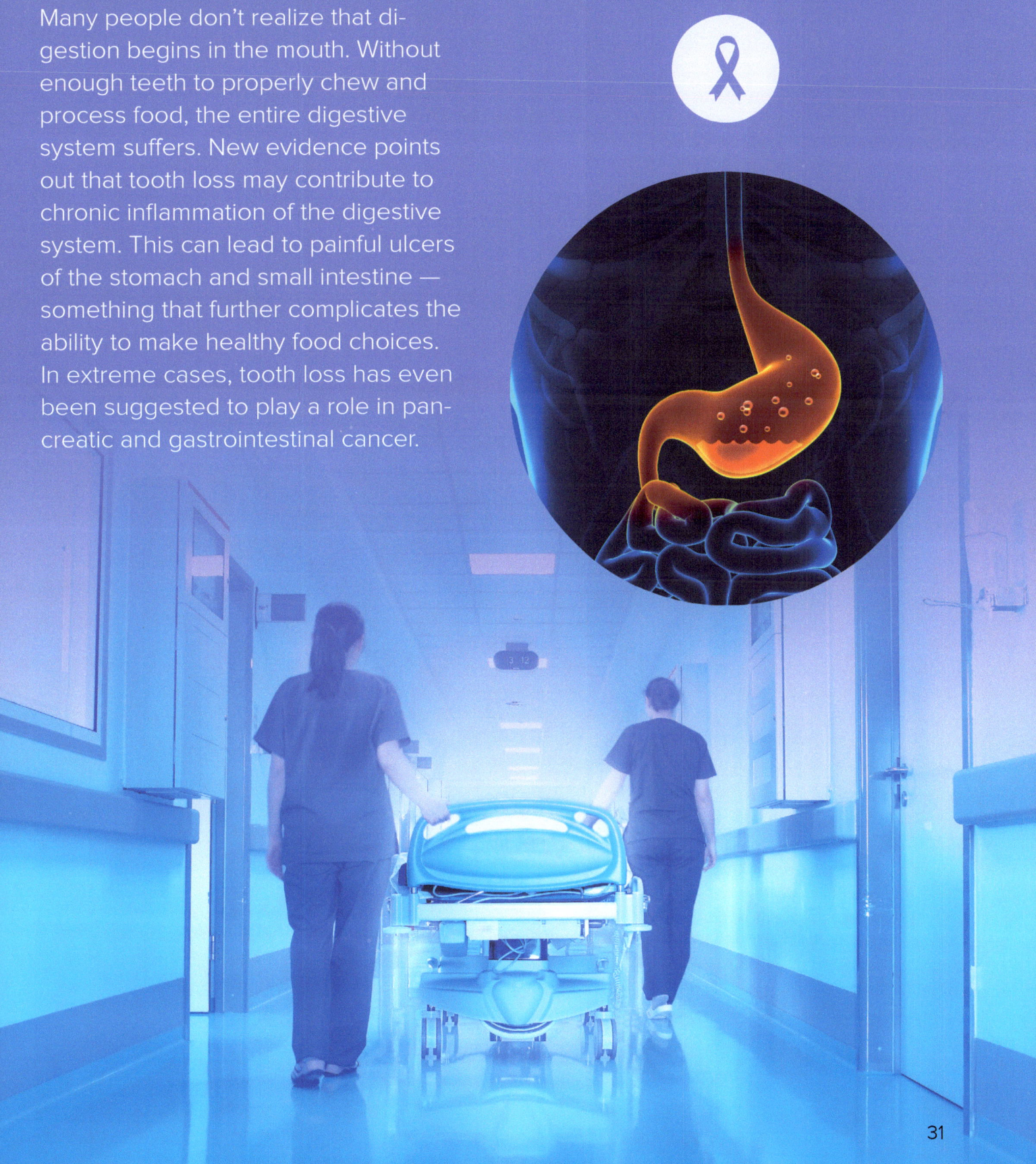

Avoid the sugar rush

As you can imagine — a diet high in fat, cholesterol and carbohydrates (soft easy to eat foods) lends itself to obesity and diabetes. A study carried out in New York in 1995 suggested that patients who had experienced tooth loss were at a higher risk of diabetes and obesity.

Tooth loss and its consequences has been linked to obesity and non-insulin dependent diabetes.

Living with a Heavy Heart

According to the CDC, heart disease is the leading cause of death. Heart disease kills more people every year than lung disease, the flu, accidents, Alzheimers and diabetes combined. So it's important to understand all of the reasons one may develop heart problems. One of the causes is tooth loss. A 2010 study carried out in a Swedish university suggested that the number of teeth remaining may be a predictor for risk of death from heart disease. Here is a list of heart issues linked to tooth loss:

1. **Electrocardiographic abnormalities**

2. **High blood pressure**

3. **Heart failure**

4. **Ischemic heart disease**

5. **Stroke**

6. **Aortic valve sclerosis**

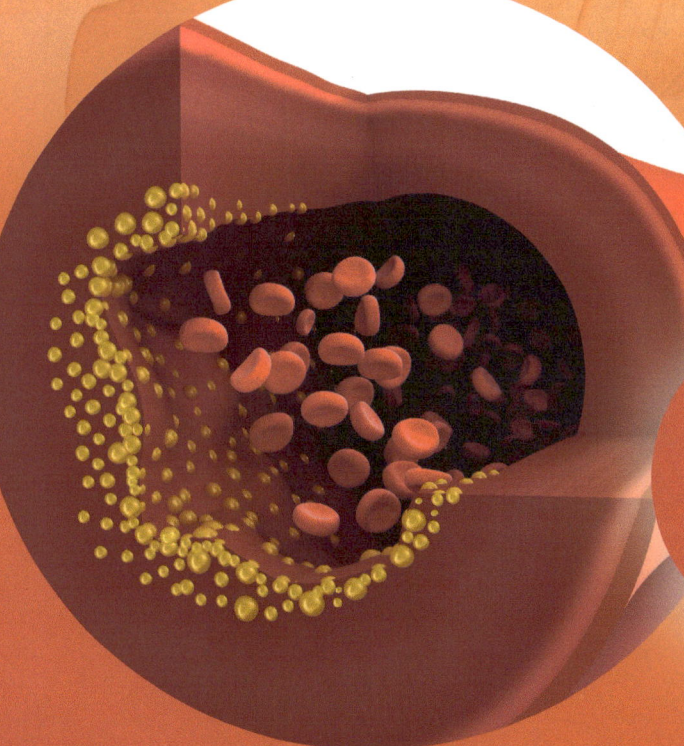

Here you can see a blood vessel getting narrower from cholesterol buildup.

Heart disease kills more people every year than lung disease, the flu, accidents, Alzheimers and diabetes combined

Don't turn into a Home Body

Several studies have shown that tooth loss is associated with a lower quality of life. A study carried out in Germany showed that having a stable set of teeth "prevents the decline of daily function and improves social interaction and general well being."

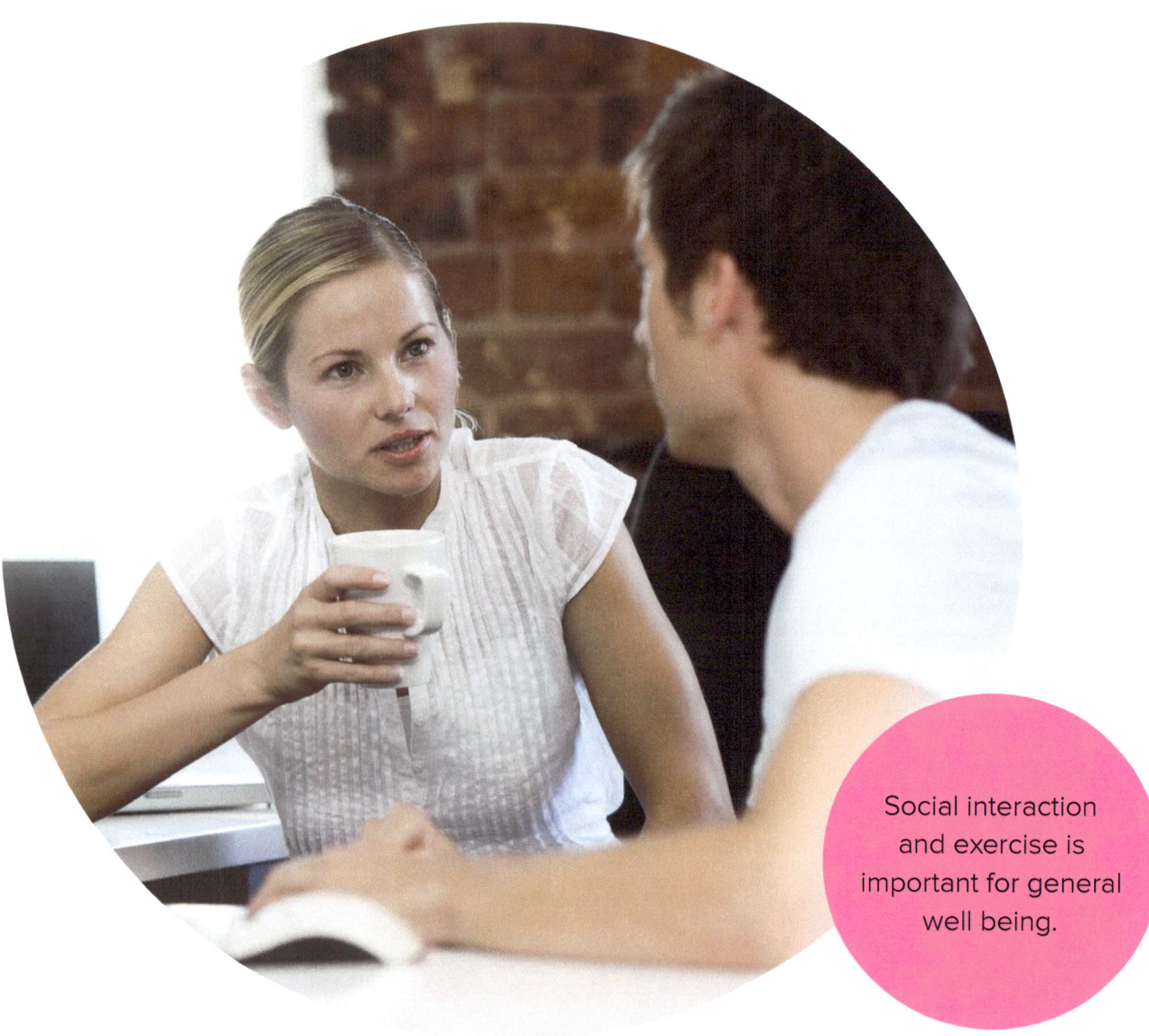

Social interaction and exercise is important for general well being.

Catch Your Breath

A study carried out in Italy shows that people who have no teeth are at a greater risk of sleep apnea – a condition in which a person doesn't breath correctly while sleeping. It can cause a lot of health problems like high blood pressure, heart disease, stroke, diabetes and depression.

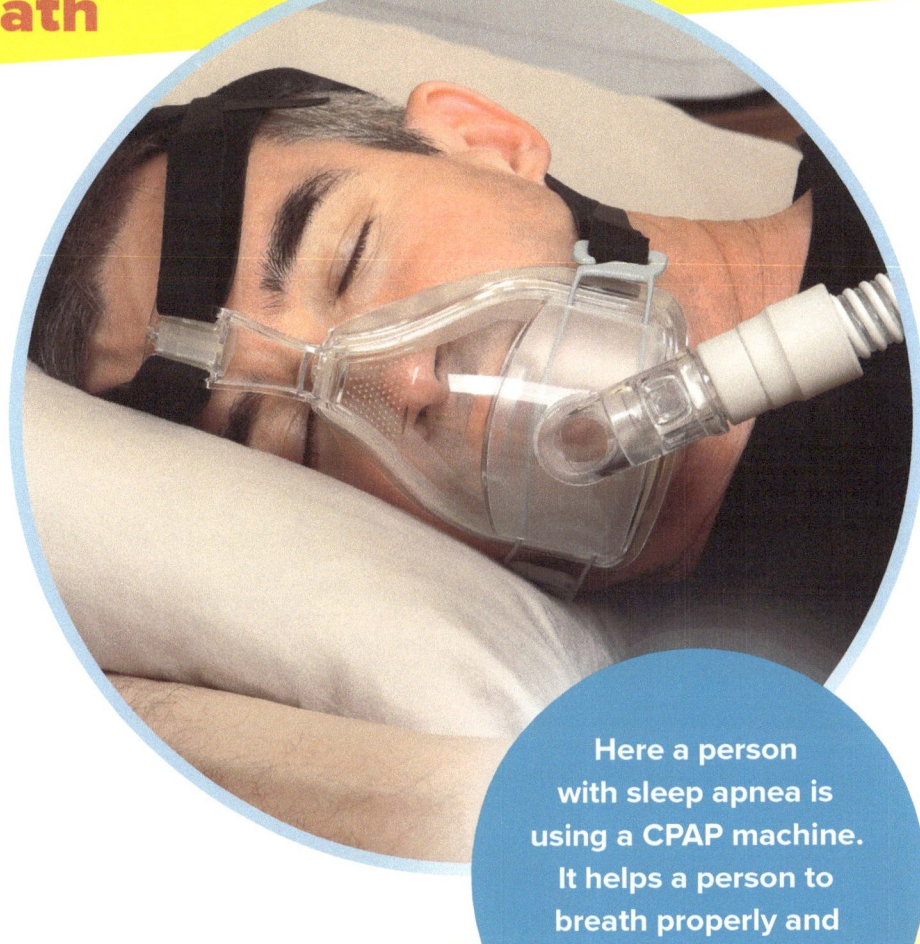

Here a person with sleep apnea is using a CPAP machine. It helps a person to breath properly and get enough oxygen during sleep.

So who should replace their teeth?

Everyone should strive to replace lost teeth. If there is one thing we know it's that tooth loss is increasingly becoming a predictor for poor health in the future. It makes complete sense. If you don't have enough teeth the digestive system becomes overloaded and the food choices you make become poor ones. A spiral effect causes your entire body to eventually get out of balance and increases chances of disease and poor health. Dental wellbeing is just one small aspect of your overall health but it can have a profound effect on the rest of your body. Luckily, today's dental patients have a myriad of options available. It's now possible to completely replace any lost teeth in a very predictable and easy way with dental implants.

the DENTAL IMPLANTS Checklist

When it comes to dental implants, there are very few true restrictions. The vast majority of people are great candidates for dental implants — a reason implant therapy has become so popular. Still, there are some important considerations for anyone ready to leap into the exciting world of implant supported teeth.

Control the sugar rush

Many patients with diabetes are successfully treated with dental implants. In fact, people who learn to control their blood sugar heal uneventfully and can be treated like anyone else. Blood sugar control is usually measured using HBA1C or Hemoglobin A1c. This is a number written on most blood test results that helps determine how well blood sugar is controlled long term. Usually, if your HBA1C is 7.5 or below, dental implants can be placed with success rates similar to those without diabetes. If your HBA1c is too high, it's important to visit your medical doctor and get it under control. Surgery is usually postponed until blood sugar is controlled to ensure predictable surgical outcomes.

Blood thinners

Unlike other blood thinners like Plavix™ or Coumadin™, you can usually continue to take baby aspirin without interruption since it usually doesn't create any issues during surgery.

Dental implant placement is a minor surgical procedure. Even so, it's important to ensure predictable blood clotting. That's why patients taking blood thinners like Coumadin™, Plavix™, Xarelta™, Pradaxa™, Eliquis™ and full size Aspirin need to speak to their doctor about stopping anticoagulant therapy prior to surgery. Sometimes patients in a high risk category need to have implants placed in a hospital setting where it is easier to control bleeding issues.

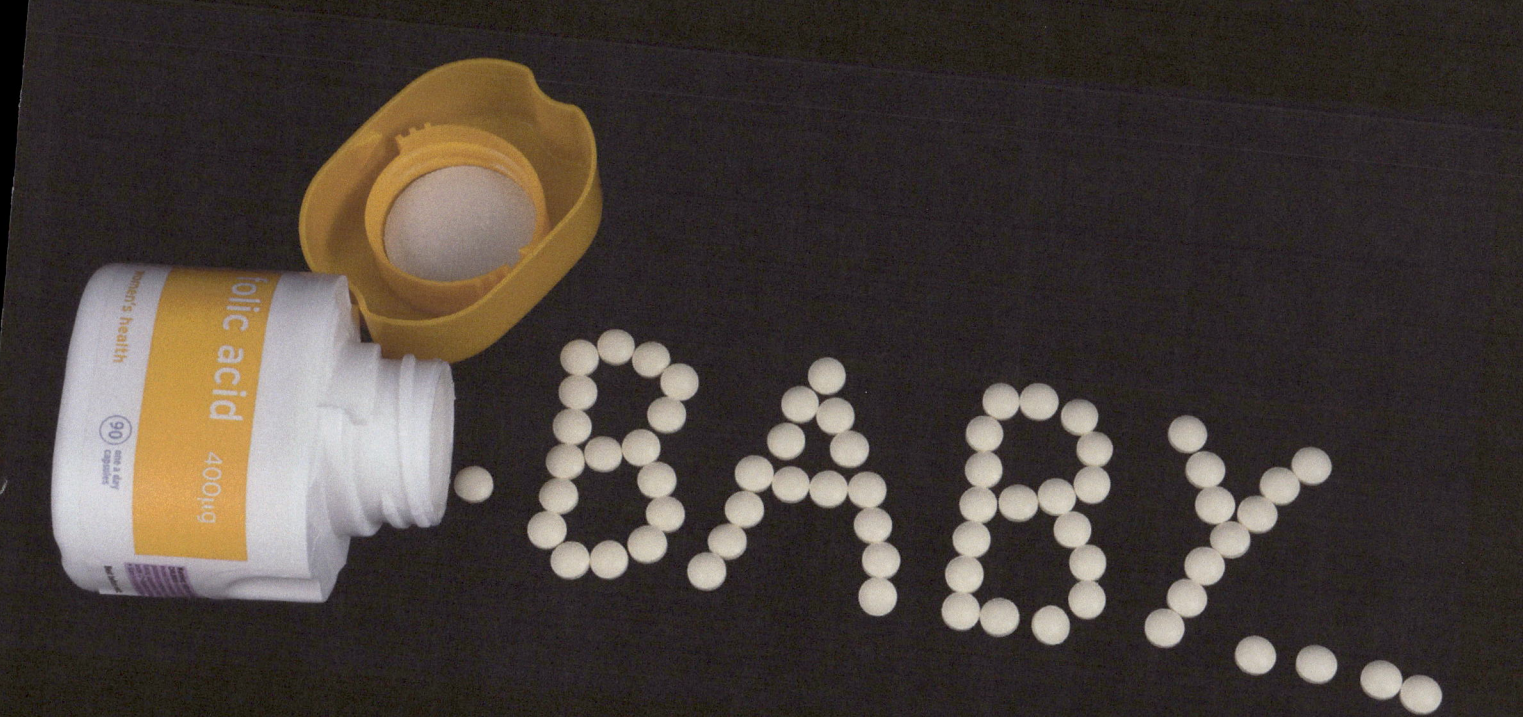

Advanced osteoporosis

While most patients who have osteoporosis can enjoy dental implant therapy, those who have taken Bisphosphonate medications like Fosamax™ or Boniva™ for longer than 7 years may need to take special precautions.

Patients with advanced osteoporosis who receive IV bisphosphonate injections are often not candidates for dental implants because of the way their bone heals. This applies to a small percent of people with very advanced osteoporosis.

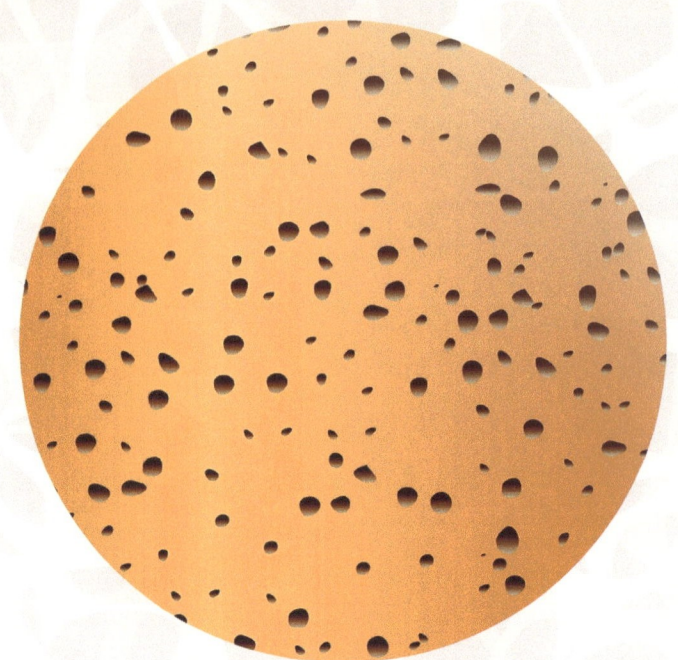

NORMAL BONE

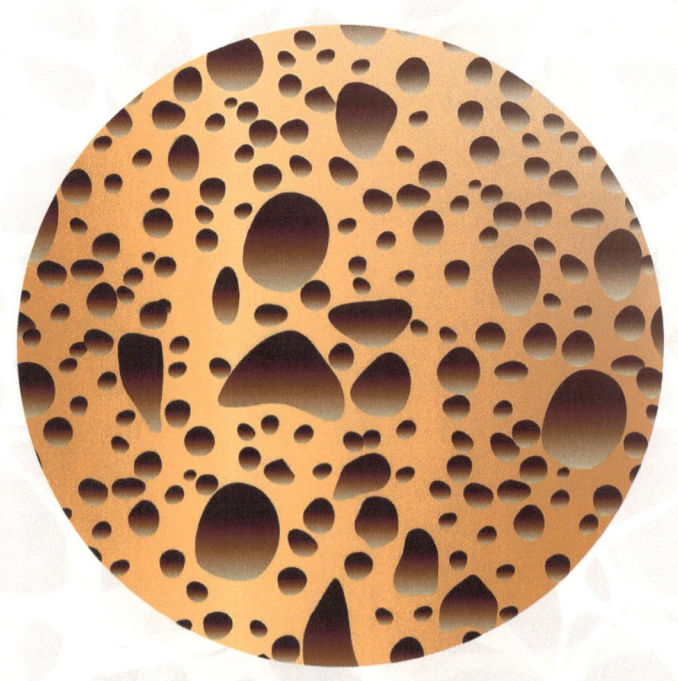

OSTEOPOROSIS

Various Health Conditions

Recent major surgery or other serious health issues may be a reason to temporarily avoid implant surgery. Patients who have a complex medical history often need a team approach to dental implant therapy. This means that the medical and dental professionals work closely to ensure a successful treatment outcome.

Controlling the bugs

For most dental implant surgeries, antibiotics are a good idea. Though the difference they make on success rate is not staggering, there is definitely a reason to use them. The statistics show that out of about 33 implants, 1 will not integrate if antibiotics are excluded. This may seem like odds that aren't worth taking a pill three times a day for a week until you think about it a different way: what if YOU are the 1 out of 33. Doing anything that improves your chance of success is worth doing. Antibiotics are especially important for dental implant surgeries involving the removal of teeth or bone grafting.

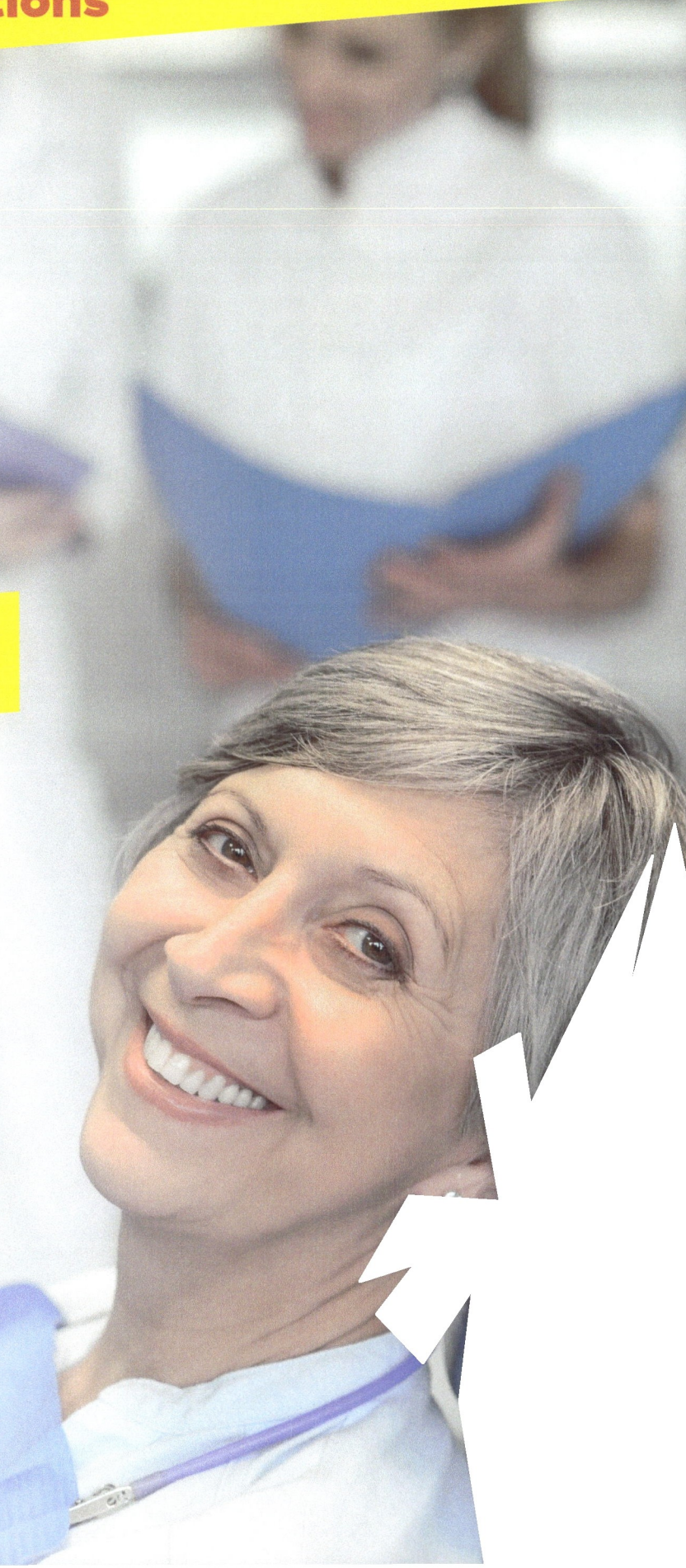

AFTER SURGERY
A list of instructions

After you undergo dental implant surgery, you'll find that in most cases the amount of discomfort that you experience is minimal and the healing process is uneventful. To ensure the most predictable and successful experience, there are a few things that you should consider:

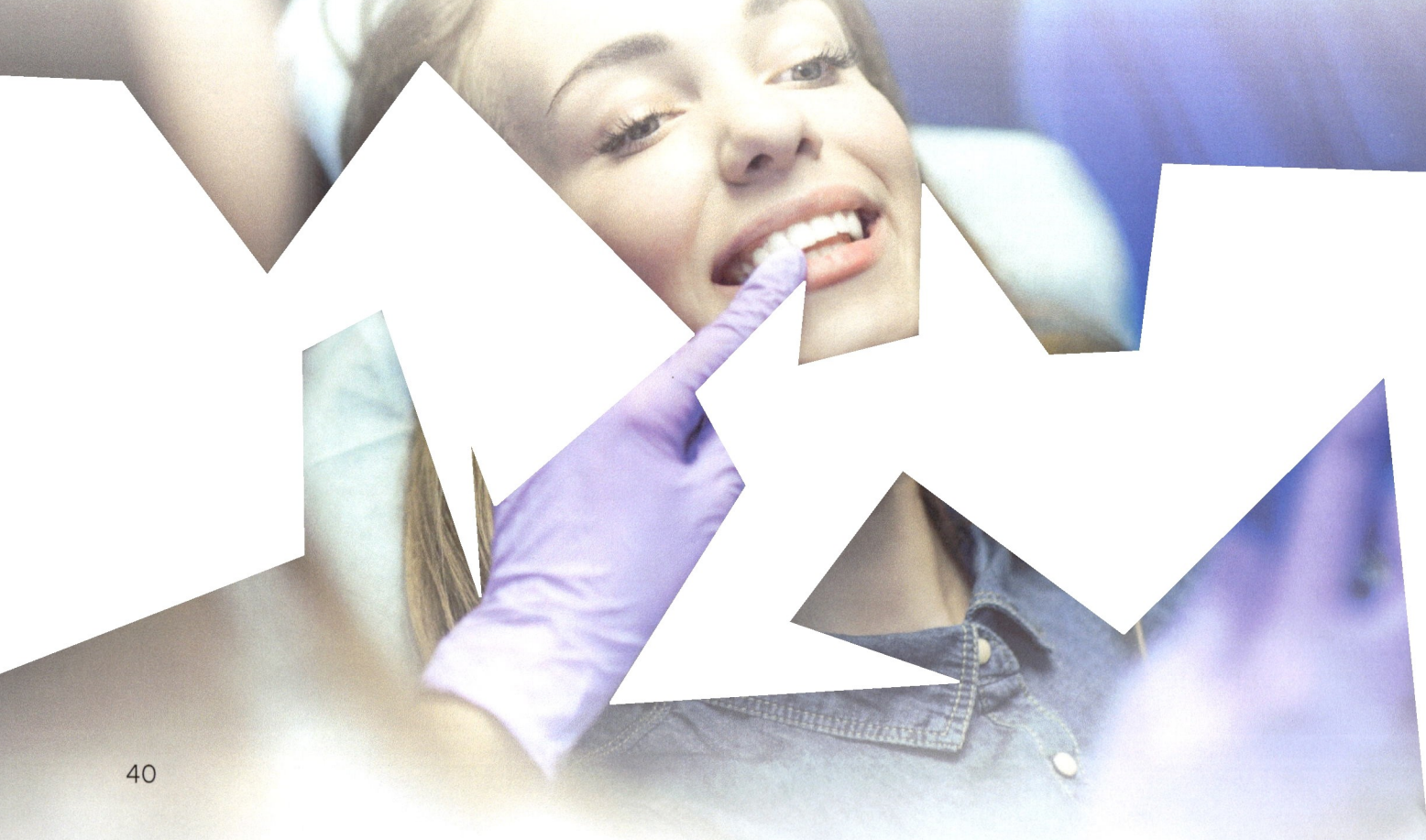

Oozing is ok

Slight bleeding is normal following implant surgery and may persist until the next day. Immediately after surgery, use mild pressure with moist gauze over the surgical site for the next two hours. DO NOT rinse or spit. Later, if bleeding becomes a problem, apply moist gauze with pressure for 15 minutes and repeat if necessary. If you don't have any gauze consider using a tea bag. Simply place it over the surgical area and gently bite down. Tea leaves naturally contain tannic acid that is known to help in bleeding control.

Why am I bleeding so much?

Remember that some oozing around the surgical area is completely normal for up to two days after surgery. Don't worry if you see a lot of red. In most cases very little blood is actually coming out – it's mostly saliva or spit that has mixed with a bit of blood.

Biting on a moist tea bag helps to stop bleeding. Replace the tea bag every 15 minutes until bleeding stops.

Things to avoid on the day of surgery

- Avoid hot or spicy food and beverages.

- Strenuous activity like exercising or lifting heavy objects the day of the surgery

- Smoking which can cause dry socket and significantly hamper the healing process.

- Drinking alcohol since alcohol is a blood thinner and can increase your chances of bleeding

Keep up the hygiene

You can gently rinse the day after surgery in order to promote healing and maintain cleanliness. Use Chlorhexidine rinse twice a day at morning and evening (2 to 3 times a day). You can gently rinse your mouth with warm salt water (teaspoon of salt in a cup of warm water). Avoid commercial mouthwashes and remember to gently brush and floss the rest of your mouth as usual.

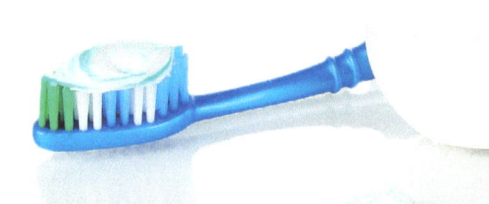

What about pain?

Ibuprofen

$C_{13}H_{18}O_2$

CH_3

CH_3

OH

In most cases, Ibuprofen is all a person needs to control discomfort following surgery. Ibuprofen is preferred to other analgesics because of its anti-inflammatory properties.

Following surgery, it is normal to experience some discomfort. In most cases, 400-600mg of Ibuprofen taken every 6-8 hours will control the pain and inflammation. If Ibuprofen alone is not providing enough relief, consider taking Ibuprofen and Tylenol™ (Acetaminophen) at the same time. Since they are processed differently, it's ok to take them simultaneously. Narcotic pain medication is usually unnecessary.

What about swelling?

Using an ice pack every 15 to 20 minutes for the first 24 hours after surgery can help to minimize swelling and increase comfort. This is especially important if teeth were removed or bone grafting material was placed during dental implant surgery.

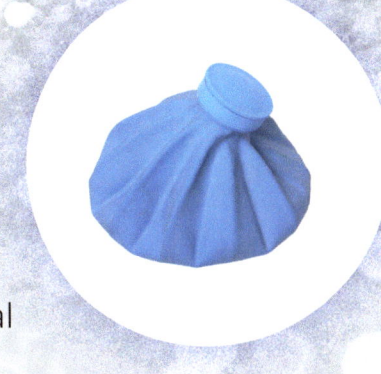

If your dental implant surgery involved the removal of a lot of teeth or bone grafting, you can expect some swelling. Note that swelling is part of the healing process and it will reach it's maximum on the second or third day after surgery. It may take more than a week for swelling to eventually subside. This is completely normal. To minimize swelling, apply an ice bag for 20 minutes and then take it off for 20 minutes the day of the surgery. After the first day, ice will not make much of a difference. If you have some difficulty opening your mouth after surgery don't worry. It will pass as the inflammation decreases. In the rare instance that you develop substantial bruising, notify the dentist who may decide to prescribe a steroid.

Keep on eating

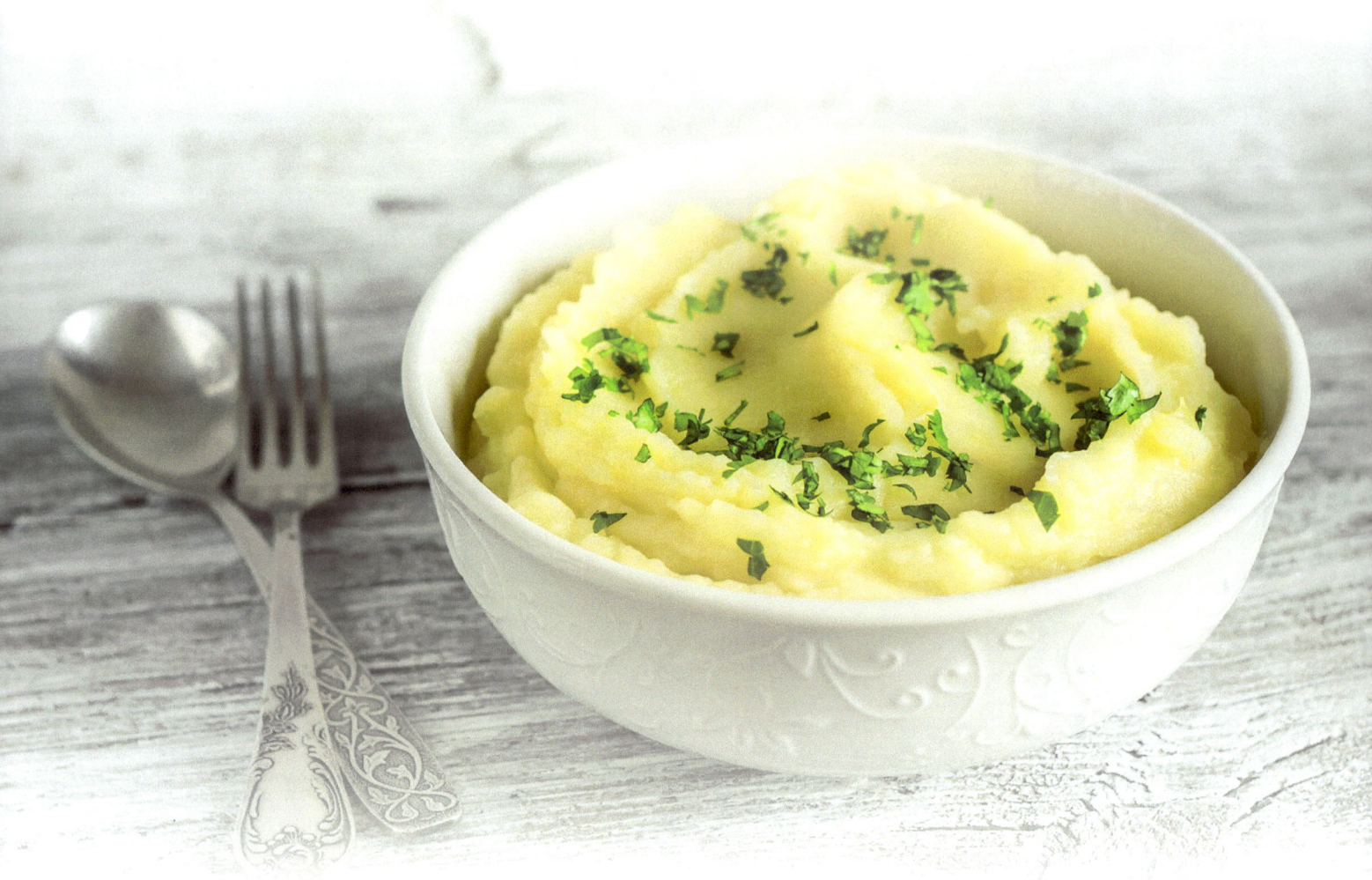

Make sure to continue taking in food and fluids. Soft nutrient rich food like mashed potatoes, soup and smoothies are a good choice while the healing process takes place. Avoid hot or spicy food immediately after surgery since it can irritate the surgical site.

Food and fluid intake is important for your wellbeing. Chewing may be difficult at first so start with soft foods and nourishing liquids. Slowly add in harder foods as healing continues. Do not use straws for the first few days after surgery and avoid anything grainy that could get stuck in the healing wound.

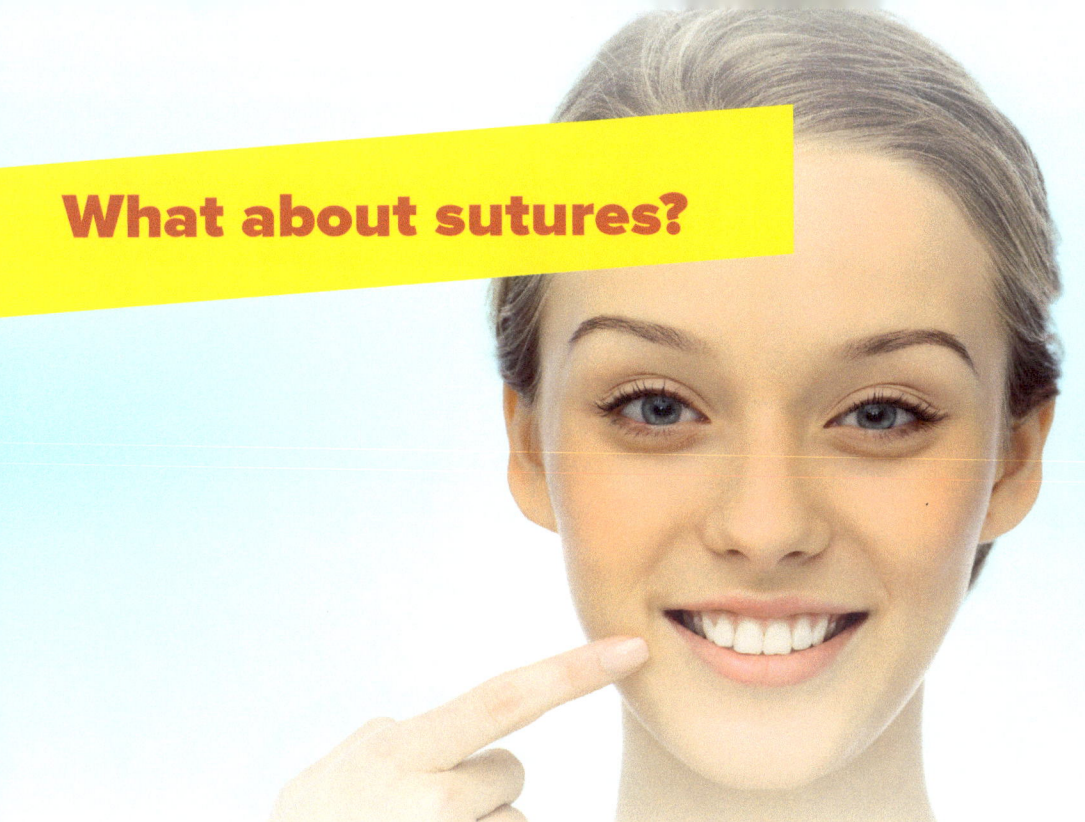

What about sutures?

It depends on the types of sutures that were used during surgery. Today, most surgery involves sutures that naturally dissolve after about 2 weeks. However, in some cases non-dissolving sutures may be used which will require a follow up appointment for suture removal. In most cases suture removal is quick and painless.

What if my implant doesn't integrate?

This is the most common question people ask and a major concern for almost all dental implant patients. The first thing you have to understand is that the odds are in your favor. In most cases, 99% of implants for bottom teeth integrate successfully and 95% of implants placed for top teeth integrate without any issues. So for the vast majority of people — this is never an issue. Of course there is that small percentage that unfortunately experiences implant failure. In this case the implant that hasn't integrated is gently removed and the area cleaned. Then another implant is either placed into the same area or next to it. It is very rare to have a dental implant not integrate the second time — the second time around they are almost always successful.

What if I am allergic to Penicillin?

Since taking an antibiotic is an important element of the protocol for dental implant surgery, people allergic to penicillin can be prescribed a different antibiotic such as clindamycin.

FINAL THOUGHTS

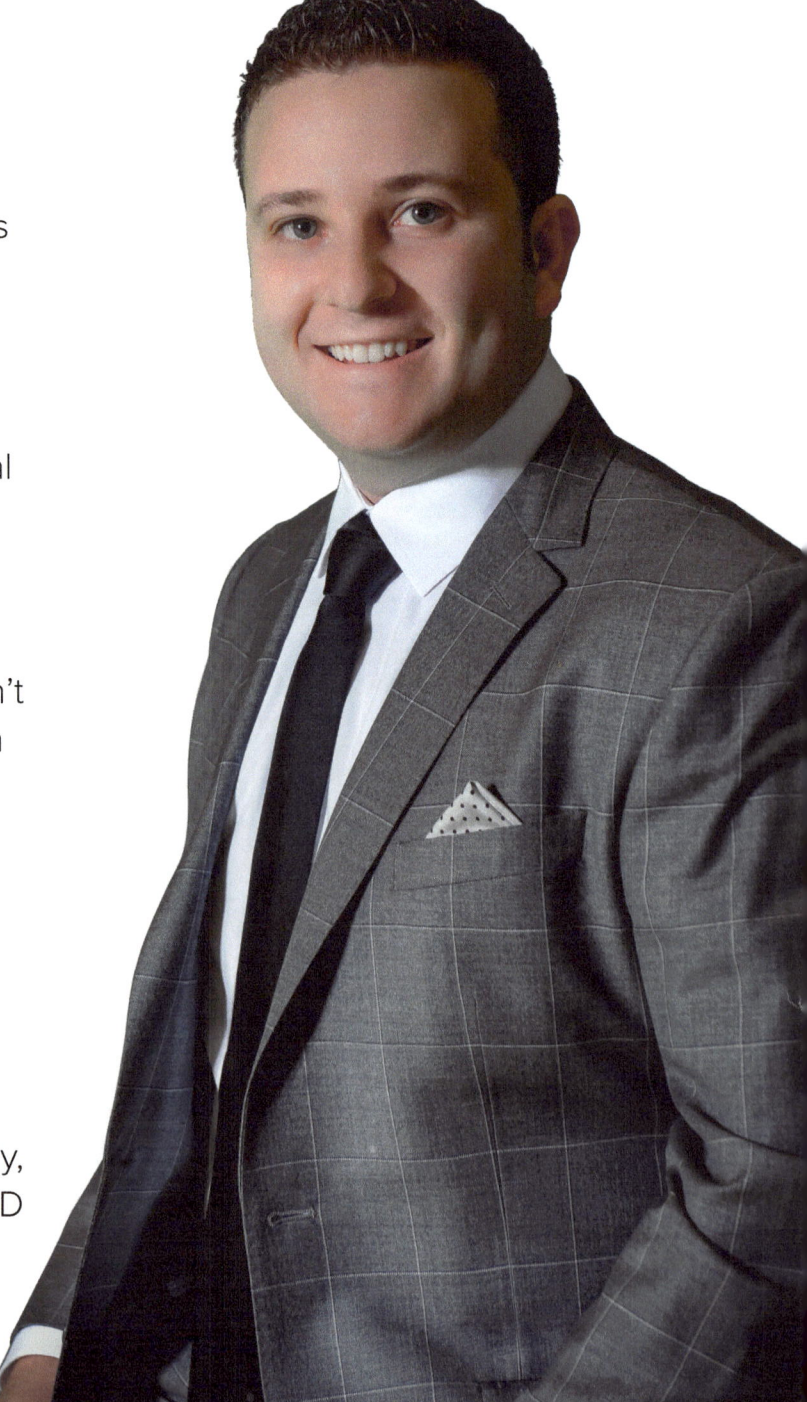

It is my sincere hope that this book has been useful and provided information and ideas that change your life for the better. Those interested in dental implants should feel confident that an option exists to ensure a stable, natural result that stands the test of time.

Whether you end up with an implant supported denture or a completely fixed bridge on several implants doesn't matter. All that matters is that you learn to love your smile and use it to it's full potential.

Yours Truly,
Maxim Babiner DMD

www.ingramcontent.com/pod-product-compliance
Lightning Source LLC
Chambersburg PA
CBHW041520280526
45792CB00004B/1321